Independent PMHNP-BC Exam Study Guide 2027-2028:

700 Practice Questions, Expert Rationales & Complete Domain Coverage for Psychiatric Mental Health NP

Caldwell Abiodun

Author Introduction

The Psychiatric Mental Health Nurse Practitioner (PMHNP) certification represents a critical standard within advanced practice nursing, reflecting the growing demand for highly skilled clinicians capable of addressing complex mental health needs across diverse populations. This field integrates clinical expertise, evidence-based psychiatric care, and holistic patient management within a rapidly evolving healthcare landscape.

The author of this study resource brings extensive subject-matter expertise in advanced nursing practice, with a focused emphasis on psychiatric and mental health care competencies aligned with national certification standards. The development of this guide is grounded in a systematic analysis of official exam content outlines, ensuring comprehensive coverage of diagnostic frameworks, psychopharmacology, therapeutic modalities, and patient-centered care strategies. Each domain has been carefully structured to reflect the cognitive demands and clinical reasoning expectations required for entry into advanced psychiatric practice.

The material reflects a disciplined methodology that prioritizes clarity, accuracy, and applied understanding. Complex clinical concepts are presented through structured explanations that reinforce diagnostic reasoning, treatment planning, and ethical decision-making. Particular attention has been given to integrating current clinical guidelines, DSM-based diagnostic criteria, and interdisciplinary care principles. Content has undergone multiple stages of editorial review to ensure consistency, technical precision, and alignment with professional standards expected of nurse practitioners.

Quality assurance processes include cross-referencing with established psychiatric nursing competencies and validation against commonly tested knowledge areas. The author's approach emphasizes not only content mastery but also the development of critical thinking skills necessary for real-world clinical application. This ensures that learners are prepared to navigate both examination scenarios and professional practice environments with confidence.

This guide is positioned as an independent educational resource designed to support candidates in their preparation for PMHNP certification. It reflects a commitment to advancing professional competence, supporting lifelong learning, and contributing to the delivery of safe, effective, and evidence-based mental health care.

Table of Contents

Copyright

This guide is not affiliated with the American Nurses Credentialing Center (ANCC) or any governing body. The ANCC name and exam title are used solely to denote alignment with the publicly available test content outline. The content herein is intended to support graduate-level learners, clinical educators, and certification candidates by providing structured study material that accurately represents the scope of knowledge required for board certification.

The 2026 edition integrates updates in psychiatric nursing science, pharmacology, psychotherapy models, and health ethics to reflect the evolving standards of advanced practice. The author and compiler acknowledge that all material builds upon recognized nursing and medical scholarship, interpreted and paraphrased for clarity and synthesis within a professional educational context.

Disclaimer

Chapter 1: Scientific Foundation

The scientific foundation domain establishes the biological, physiological, and developmental underpinnings of psychiatric nursing. It provides the conceptual and evidence-based framework for interpreting mental illness as an interaction of neurobiology, genetics, pharmacodynamics, and psychosocial influences. A psychiatric–mental health nurse practitioner must demonstrate not only factual knowledge of the nervous system but also the ability to apply it to patient assessment, medication management, and interdisciplinary collaboration.

The study of advanced pathophysiology connects the biological mechanisms of disease with observable clinical symptoms. Within psychiatric care, this involves understanding how alterations in neurotransmitter pathways, receptor sensitivity, endocrine balance, and inflammatory processes affect behavior, emotion, and cognition. The PMHNP applies this foundation when distinguishing psychiatric symptoms from physiological conditions that mimic or contribute to them—for example, differentiating thyroid dysfunction from major depressive disorder or delirium from psychosis.

Advanced pharmacology deepens this biological perspective by linking drug mechanisms to neural function. The practitioner must grasp how medications act at synaptic and systemic levels, recognizing interactions, contraindications, and the significance of pharmacogenomics. Gene–drug interactions can modify response to antidepressants or antipsychotics, requiring precise titration and vigilant monitoring.

A comprehensive understanding of neurodevelopment is critical for lifespan mental health assessment. The developing brain undergoes periods of vulnerability and plasticity; early stress, trauma, or exposure to toxins can alter synaptic pruning, myelination, and neurotransmitter regulation. These changes underlie many psychiatric disorders that emerge later in life. For example, disruptions in the hypothalamic–pituitary–adrenal (HPA) axis during childhood can predispose individuals to anxiety or mood dysregulation in adulthood.

Neuroanatomy and Neurophysiology

The central nervous system, composed of the brain and spinal cord, orchestrates mental function through complex networks of neurons and glial cells. Each region contributes uniquely to cognition, emotion, and behavior. The **frontal lobe** governs executive function, impulse control, and emotional regulation—areas frequently affected in mood and personality disorders. The **limbic system**, encompassing the amygdala, hippocampus, and cingulate gyrus, integrates memory with affective processing and is central to understanding trauma-related and anxiety disorders.

Neurophysiological processes depend on the dynamic exchange of ions and neurotransmitters. Communication between neurons occurs at synapses, where electrical impulses trigger the release of chemical messengers such as serotonin, dopamine, gamma-aminobutyric acid (GABA), and glutamate. Each neurotransmitter system has a distinctive role: dopamine regulates motivation and reward, serotonin modulates mood and sleep, GABA produces inhibitory control, and glutamate drives excitatory signaling essential for cognition. Dysregulation within or between these systems contributes to clinical syndromes like schizophrenia, depression, and bipolar disorder.

Psychopharmacology and Pharmacodynamics

Psychopharmacology extends from neurophysiology, explaining how medications influence neuronal communication. The PMHNP must interpret the mechanisms of action for major drug classes, including antidepressants, antipsychotics, anxiolytics, mood stabilizers, and stimulants. Medications may act as **agonists**, enhancing receptor activity, or **antagonists**, blocking neurotransmitter binding.

Pharmacodynamics describes the biochemical interaction between drug and receptor, whereas pharmacokinetics addresses absorption, distribution, metabolism, and excretion. For instance, selective serotonin reuptake inhibitors (SSRIs) increase serotonin availability by inhibiting its reuptake transporter, while mood stabilizers such as lithium modulate intracellular signaling cascades to stabilize affective states.

Genetic polymorphisms in enzymes such as CYP2D6 and CYP2C19 influence individual response to psychotropic agents. The application of pharmacogenomic testing exemplifies precision mental health care—allowing the practitioner to anticipate metabolic variations and optimize dosing.

Neurodevelopment and Lifespan Considerations

Human neurodevelopment follows a sequence of growth, differentiation, and pruning that extends from prenatal life into the third decade. Understanding this trajectory allows the PMHNP to contextualize psychiatric symptoms within the appropriate developmental stage. Synaptic density peaks in early childhood, then refines through selective elimination—a process shaped by genetics and environmental experience. Excessive pruning in adolescence has been associated with schizophrenia, while deficient pruning may contribute to neurodevelopmental disorders such as autism spectrum disorder.

Prenatal exposure to stress, infection, or toxins alters neural migration and cortical connectivity. For instance, maternal stress during the second trimester may elevate fetal cortisol levels, sensitizing the infant's stress response system. The concept of **neuroplasticity** underscores that the brain remains capable of structural and functional adaptation throughout life, supporting recovery through psychotherapy, pharmacologic modulation, and lifestyle interventions.

Lifespan care demands recognition of how neurobiology interacts with age-related changes. Pediatric populations require medication dosing calibrated to immature hepatic metabolism and evolving receptor sensitivity, while geriatric patients experience decreased renal clearance and increased blood–brain barrier permeability. The PMHNP uses these insights to minimize adverse effects and tailor therapeutic regimens.

Psychogenomics and Individual Variation

Psychogenomics integrates genetic, epigenetic, and pharmacologic science to explain how inherited traits influence psychiatric vulnerability and medication response. Variants in genes regulating serotonin transport (5-HTTLPR), dopamine receptors (DRD2, DRD4), and neurotrophic factors (BDNF) correlate with emotional regulation and resilience to stress. Environmental factors—trauma, nutrition, or substance exposure—can modify gene expression without altering the DNA sequence through **epigenetic mechanisms** such as methylation or histone modification.

In clinical application, the PMHNP interprets pharmacogenomic panels to adjust drug selection and dosing. For instance, patients who are poor metabolizers of CYP2D6 substrates may require reduced dosages of tricyclic antidepressants to avoid toxicity. Similarly, those with polymorphisms affecting serotonin transport may show variable response to SSRIs. The integration of genomic data into psychiatric care exemplifies the movement toward personalized medicine, ensuring efficacy while reducing trial-and-error prescribing.

Genomic awareness also enhances risk prediction. A family history of mood or psychotic disorders reflects polygenic inheritance rather than single-gene causation, demanding careful family assessment and preventive counseling. By interpreting these patterns, the PMHNP functions as a clinician–scientist, merging molecular insight with therapeutic judgment.

Advanced Physical Assessment

The ability to perform a comprehensive and focused physical examination distinguishes advanced practice from general nursing. Psychiatric assessment extends beyond mental status evaluation to include systemic review. Neurological signs, endocrine disturbances, or medication side effects often manifest as psychiatric symptoms. An example is the appearance of agitation or cognitive impairment secondary to metabolic imbalance or medication interaction.

The PMHNP employs advanced techniques of inspection, palpation, percussion, and auscultation, integrating findings into the psychiatric context. Assessment of vital signs, endocrine function, cardiovascular status, and neurologic reflexes supports accurate differential diagnosis. A thorough medication history is vital to distinguish adverse effects such as extrapyramidal symptoms or serotonin syndrome from primary psychiatric pathology.

Integrating Biological and Psychological Models

The modern PMHNP applies an integrative framework linking biological substrates to psychological experience. This biopsychosocial model recognizes that emotional suffering reflects the interaction of neural, cognitive, and environmental processes. Biological vulnerability interacts with stress exposure, personality traits, and coping capacity. For instance, depressive disorders may arise from serotonergic dysregulation compounded by maladaptive cognitive schemas.

Through this synthesis, the nurse practitioner interprets patient presentations holistically. Treatment planning thus includes psychopharmacology, psychotherapy, and social interventions rather than isolated modalities. The scientific foundation domain equips clinicians to interpret evidence, translate research findings into practice, and articulate rationales for clinical decisions within interdisciplinary teams.

Neuroendocrinology and Stress Regulation

The endocrine system and the nervous system operate in continuous dialogue, orchestrating physiological and emotional balance. Central to this interaction is the **hypothalamic–pituitary–adrenal (HPA) axis**, a feedback loop that governs the body's response to stress. When a person perceives threat, the hypothalamus secretes corticotropin-releasing hormone (CRH), prompting the pituitary gland to release adrenocorticotropic hormone (ACTH). ACTH stimulates the adrenal cortex to produce cortisol, which mobilizes glucose, elevates cardiovascular tone, and suppresses nonessential functions.

For the PMHNP, understanding the HPA axis is essential to interpreting the biological underpinnings of anxiety, depression, and trauma. Chronic activation leads to dysregulation: cortisol levels may become persistently high or paradoxically blunted, affecting mood, immunity, and metabolism. Clinical manifestations include insomnia, fatigue, impaired concentration, and emotional volatility. Pharmacologic agents such as selective serotonin reuptake inhibitors indirectly modulate HPA activity by enhancing serotonergic inhibition of stress circuits, while mindfulness and behavioral therapies restore physiological equilibrium through parasympathetic activation.

Endocrine–psychiatric interactions extend beyond cortisol. Dysfunctions in the thyroid, adrenal, and gonadal systems frequently mimic or exacerbate psychiatric symptoms. Hypothyroidism may present as depression, while hyperthyroidism can precipitate anxiety or agitation. Estrogen fluctuations influence serotonin and dopamine levels, explaining mood changes associated with premenstrual or perimenopausal transitions. The PMHNP's advanced assessment must therefore include endocrine screening to distinguish primary psychiatric conditions from secondary hormonal disturbances.

Psychoneuroimmunology: Linking Mind, Brain, and Immunity

Psychoneuroimmunology (PNI) explores how psychological processes influence immune function. Emotional stress triggers neuroendocrine pathways that modulate immune cell activity. Persistent sympathetic arousal elevates inflammatory cytokines—interleukin-6, tumor necrosis factor-alpha, and C-reactive protein—contributing to the pathophysiology of depression and anxiety.

Conversely, supportive social interaction, positive affect, and therapeutic alliance enhance immune competence by reducing inflammation and promoting parasympathetic dominance. Research demonstrates that psychotherapeutic interventions can normalize immune markers, underscoring the biological validity of psychological healing. The PMHNP integrates PNI principles by encouraging stress management, adequate sleep, balanced nutrition, and regular physical activity as components of psychiatric treatment.

Inflammatory hypotheses of depression suggest that immune dysregulation alters neurotransmission through tryptophan depletion and microglial activation. Recognition of these mechanisms invites novel therapies—anti-inflammatory agents, omega-3 fatty acids, or lifestyle interventions—targeted to biological substrates of mood disturbance. Integrating such knowledge enhances comprehensive care that bridges mind and body.

Brain Imaging and Functional Research Interpretation

Modern neuroimaging technologies—MRI, fMRI, PET, and SPECT—provide visual evidence of brain activity and structural change associated with psychiatric conditions. The PMHNP interprets these findings not as diagnostic absolutes but as supportive data contextualizing symptom patterns.

Structural MRI reveals volume reductions in the hippocampus and prefrontal cortex among patients with chronic stress or major depressive disorder, while functional MRI demonstrates altered connectivity in the default mode network of individuals with schizophrenia. PET imaging using radiolabeled tracers highlights metabolic abnormalities or receptor availability, such as decreased dopamine D2 binding in substance use disorders.

Although these images provide insight into neural correlates, they do not define the person. The PMHNP integrates imaging results with clinical observation, avoiding deterministic interpretations. Brain imaging strengthens biological literacy and supports patient education, helping individuals visualize how therapy and medication foster tangible neurobiological recovery. Understanding this research also positions the practitioner to interpret emerging literature critically and translate evidence into practice.

Behavioral Genetics and Heritability of Mental Disorders

Behavioral genetics examines the contribution of inherited factors to psychiatric vulnerability. Twin and adoption studies consistently show heritability estimates: schizophrenia (~80%), bipolar disorder (~70%), and major depressive disorder (~40%). Yet genetics confer probability, not destiny. Environmental moderators—trauma, stress, nutrition—shape gene expression through epigenetic mechanisms.

The PMHNP explains to patients that family history indicates risk, not inevitability. Genetic predisposition interacts with resilience factors such as social support, cognitive flexibility, and meaning-making. Genetic counseling may be appropriate for families concerned about transmission of severe mental illness, ensuring understanding without stigma.

Molecular genetics continues to identify susceptibility loci—COMT variants affecting dopamine degradation, DISC1 associated with neurodevelopment, and BDNF influencing neuroplasticity. These discoveries refine pharmacologic prediction models but require cautious interpretation until validated across populations. The advanced practitioner maintains awareness of evolving research, applying findings ethically and compassionately.

Neuroplasticity and Learning

Neuroplasticity—the brain's capacity to reorganize synaptic connections in response to experience—is the biological foundation for psychotherapy and recovery. Learning, memory, and behavior change rely on strengthening or weakening synaptic pathways through long-term potentiation and depression. Repetition of adaptive thoughts and behaviors consolidates new neural networks, a process visualized in studies showing hippocampal growth following cognitive-behavioral therapy for depression.

The PMHNP leverages neuroplasticity by integrating behavioral activation, mindfulness, and skill rehearsal into care plans. These interventions literally reshape neural patterns, reinforcing adaptive coping. Pharmacologic agents such as SSRIs and ketamine enhance neuroplastic potential by stimulating BDNF production, facilitating recovery from emotional trauma.

Understanding neuroplasticity transforms the practitioner's outlook: mental illness is not fixed but malleable. By framing treatment as a process of brain retraining, clinicians instill hope and agency, aligning biological science with the art of healing.

Sleep–Wake Regulation and Circadian Biology

Sleep sustains mental and physical health through synaptic homeostasis, hormonal balance, and emotional processing. The **suprachiasmatic nucleus (SCN)** in the hypothalamus functions as the master circadian pacemaker, synchronizing physiological rhythms with the light–dark cycle. Disturbances in circadian alignment manifest as mood instability, cognitive impairment, and metabolic dysfunction.

The PMHNP assesses sleep patterns as a vital sign of psychiatric health. Insomnia often precedes mood episodes, while hypersomnia may accompany atypical depression. Shift work, screen exposure, and irregular schedules desynchronize the circadian system, necessitating behavioral and pharmacologic correction.

Melatonin, secreted by the pineal gland, regulates sleep onset, while orexin neurons in the hypothalamus sustain wakefulness. Dysregulation contributes to disorders such as narcolepsy or delayed sleep phase syndrome. Treatment strategies include cognitive behavioral therapy for insomnia, sleep hygiene education, and, when appropriate, pharmacologic support with hypnotics or melatonin receptor agonists.

Sleep also mediates emotional consolidation. REM sleep integrates affective memories, whereas deprivation heightens amygdala reactivity and anxiety. By prioritizing sleep in care planning, the PMHNP addresses a fundamental determinant of mental stability.

Integrative Physiological Perspectives

The scientific foundation of psychiatric nursing encompasses systemic interdependence. Cardiovascular, gastrointestinal, and endocrine systems influence mental health through shared pathways of inflammation, neurotransmission, and autonomic regulation. The **gut–brain axis**, mediated by the vagus nerve and microbiota metabolites, illustrates how digestion affects mood. Diets rich in omega-3 fatty acids, fiber, and fermented foods support neurochemical balance by reducing inflammation and enhancing serotonin precursor availability.

The PMHNP adopts a holistic perspective, recognizing that psychiatric symptoms may signal systemic imbalance. Comprehensive assessment includes laboratory evaluation of metabolic markers, vitamin deficiencies, and inflammatory indices. Integrative strategies—nutritional counseling, physical activity promotion, and relaxation training—complement pharmacologic and psychotherapeutic modalities.

Scientific literacy enables the practitioner to interpret biomedical research critically, evaluate emerging treatments, and communicate complex concepts in accessible language. The synthesis of neurobiology, physiology, and psychosocial theory defines the advanced scientific foundation required for safe, effective, and compassionate psychiatric nursing.

Chapter 2: Advanced Practice Skills

Advanced practice in psychiatric–mental health nursing emphasizes assessment, clinical interviewing, risk management, and health promotion. The PMHNP combines scientific knowledge with communication skills to form therapeutic relationships and make accurate, ethical, and culturally competent decisions.

Clinical Interviewing

The clinical interview is both diagnostic and therapeutic. It elicits subjective data while establishing rapport and trust. Effective interviewing balances structure with empathy, allowing patients to express concerns in their own terms. The PMHNP uses open-ended questions to explore mood, perception, cognition, and behavior, observing nonverbal cues such as posture, eye contact, and affect congruence.

Techniques like **motivational interviewing** facilitate behavioral change by resolving ambivalence. The practitioner adopts a guiding style—expressing empathy, supporting self-efficacy, and highlighting discrepancies between goals and current behavior. This method is particularly valuable in substance use treatment, medication adherence, and lifestyle modification.

Clinical interviewing also involves assessing risk for harm. The PMHNP directly inquires about suicidal ideation, intent, and access to means, maintaining a balance between compassion and clarity. In crisis situations, interviews become instruments of stabilization—clarifying immediate needs, ensuring safety, and engaging supportive resources.

Health Promotion and Disease Prevention

Psychiatric well-being is inseparable from physical health. Advanced practice nursing integrates preventive strategies across the lifespan, promoting resilience and reducing relapse risk. Health promotion includes screening for metabolic syndrome in patients receiving antipsychotics, educating about sleep hygiene, nutrition, and exercise, and advocating for tobacco cessation.

Preventive interventions draw upon models such as the Health Belief Model and the Transtheoretical Model of Change, which explain how individuals progress through stages of readiness. By identifying a patient's stage—precontemplation, contemplation, preparation, action, or maintenance—the PMHNP tailors interventions that enhance motivation rather than impose compliance.

Community-level health promotion extends beyond individual counseling. Psychiatric nurse practitioners participate in public mental health initiatives, policy advocacy, and population-based screenings to detect depression, anxiety, and substance misuse. Preventive care recognizes that early identification of mental distress reduces chronic disability and societal burden.

Screening and Assessment Tools

Standardized tools enhance objectivity in psychiatric evaluation. The PMHNP selects instruments validated for age, culture, and clinical setting. Examples include the PHQ-9 for depression, GAD-7 for anxiety, Columbia Suicide Severity Rating Scale for suicide risk, and Vanderbilt ADHD Rating Scales for attention disorders.

Interpretation requires understanding psychometric properties such as sensitivity, specificity, and cutoff scores. Screening outcomes guide but do not replace clinical judgment. The practitioner correlates results with patient history and physical findings to form a comprehensive diagnostic impression.

Effective assessment includes cognitive testing, such as the Mini-Mental State Examination or Montreal Cognitive Assessment, particularly in older adults. These tools identify neurocognitive decline, differentiate delirium from dementia, and direct further diagnostic testing.

Mental Status Examination

The Mental Status Examination (MSE) provides a structured framework for observing and documenting psychological functioning. Components include appearance, behavior, speech, mood, affect, thought process, thought content, perception, cognition, insight, and judgment. The PMHNP learns to interpret subtle cues—psychomotor agitation, latency of speech, affective constriction, or disorganized thinking—as indicators of underlying pathology.

In practice, the MSE forms part of every patient encounter, evolving with treatment. A dynamic MSE captures response to therapy and medication, noting improvements in attention, mood stability, or insight. Precision in observation and language is critical; terms such as "tangential," "circumstantial," or "flight of ideas" must be used accurately to communicate findings among professionals.

Psychiatric Emergency Management

Psychiatric emergencies demand rapid, precise, and compassionate intervention. The PMHNP is often the first clinician to assess acute behavioral disturbances such as suicidal crises, psychosis, or violent agitation. These scenarios require mastery of both de-escalation and medical stabilization. Immediate safety takes precedence over diagnostic clarity, yet accurate triage depends on a structured approach.

The first step involves risk recognition—identifying verbal cues, affective instability, or situational stressors that suggest imminent danger. Assessment of intent, plan, and means distinguishes passive suicidal ideation from active risk. In patients with psychosis, perceptual distortions or command hallucinations may elevate risk for self-harm or aggression. Concurrent medical causes, such as delirium, hypoglycemia, or intoxication, must always be excluded.

Intervention proceeds through verbal de-escalation before considering medication or restraint. A calm tone, safe physical distance, and clear communication promote trust even in agitation. Pharmacologic strategies include short-acting benzodiazepines or antipsychotics when nonpharmacologic measures fail. Collaboration with interdisciplinary teams—social workers, security staff, and emergency physicians—ensures comprehensive management.

After stabilization, the PMHNP develops a crisis plan emphasizing follow-up, safety contracting, and environmental support. Every encounter concludes with documentation detailing risk level, interventions, and rationale. Ethical duty extends to maintaining dignity and autonomy within the least restrictive care framework, reinforcing the patient's agency in recovery.

Psychoeducation and Recovery Promotion

Psychoeducation empowers patients and families by translating psychiatric concepts into understandable language. The PMHNP acts as an educator, helping individuals recognize symptoms, treatment options, and lifestyle factors influencing mental health. Effective teaching involves adapting communication to literacy level, cultural background, and emotional readiness.

Topics frequently addressed include medication adherence, recognition of relapse warning signs, coping mechanisms, and stress management. Psychoeducation extends beyond instruction; it fosters collaboration. Patients who understand the purpose and expected effects of medications are more likely to adhere to treatment and report side effects early.

Recovery-oriented care views the patient as an active participant rather than a passive recipient. The PMHNP encourages goal setting and celebrates incremental progress. Resilience-building strategies—mindfulness, journaling, exercise, and structured social engagement—support long-term stability. In chronic mental illness, recovery emphasizes functionality and quality of life rather than symptom eradication.

Family involvement amplifies recovery. Education of caregivers reduces stigma, enhances adherence, and mitigates caregiver burden. The practitioner's skill lies in facilitating honest communication while maintaining confidentiality. Through empathy and clear boundaries, the PMHNP sustains therapeutic alliance even amid conflict or relapse.

Risk Assessment

Risk assessment is an ongoing process that evaluates threats to safety and well-being across physical, psychological, and social domains. In psychiatric practice, the most critical risks involve suicide, homicide, and neglect. Systematic evaluation requires both structured tools and clinical judgment.

The **Columbia Suicide Severity Rating Scale** or **Beck Scale for Suicide Ideation** provides standardized metrics, but interpretation must consider context—recent loss, substance use, or hopelessness significantly elevate danger. The PMHNP evaluates protective factors such as family support, spirituality, and problem-solving ability to balance risk formulation.

Homicide risk assessment parallels this approach, focusing on intent, target specificity, access to weapons, and history of violence. In both scenarios, documentation and communication are paramount. If risk exceeds safe limits, duty-to-warn and involuntary commitment laws may apply, requiring knowledge of state statutes and institutional policy.

Neglect and self-care deficits—especially among older adults or cognitively impaired individuals—warrant assessment of functional capacity, nutritional intake, and environmental safety. Interdisciplinary collaboration with case managers and occupational therapists supports holistic care. Risk assessment culminates not in prediction but prevention, guiding timely intervention.

Substance Use Screening and Withdrawal Management

Substance use complicates psychiatric assessment and treatment. The PMHNP employs screening tools such as the AUDIT (Alcohol Use Disorders Identification Test), DAST, and CAGE questionnaire to detect problematic use. Comprehensive assessment addresses quantity, frequency, pattern, and consequences of use.

Withdrawal syndromes—whether alcohol, benzodiazepine, or opioid—require prompt recognition. Instruments such as the CIWA-Ar for alcohol and COWS for opioids quantify severity and guide pharmacologic management. The nurse practitioner monitors vital signs, tremors, and autonomic instability, adjusting medication dosages to maintain safety.

Integration of addiction science within psychiatric care supports dual-diagnosis treatment. Motivational enhancement, contingency management, and medication-assisted therapy—such as buprenorphine for opioid dependence—are critical tools. Stigma reduction and harm-reduction education empower patients to reengage with care rather than retreat into secrecy.

Integration of Recovery and Resilience Frameworks

Advanced practice integrates resilience-based models that focus on strengths rather than deficits. Resilience arises from adaptability, purpose, and social connection. The PMHNP cultivates resilience through cognitive reframing, supportive relationships, and structured activity. Interventions such as strengths-based assessment shift the narrative from illness to capacity.

Community engagement enhances recovery, offering social identity and belonging. Group therapy, peer support, and vocational rehabilitation promote autonomy. The practitioner fosters a therapeutic milieu emphasizing hope, responsibility, and empowerment—principles central to psychiatric nursing philosophy.

Therapeutic Communication and the Science of Interaction

Therapeutic communication is the foundation of every effective nurse–patient relationship. For the PMHNP, communication transcends verbal exchange; it becomes a diagnostic instrument and an intervention in itself. The practitioner applies active listening, reflection, summarization, and clarification to guide dialogue while assessing cognitive coherence, affective tone, and insight. Each encounter offers data: word choice may reveal anxiety, while silence may indicate depression or mistrust.

Neuroscientific evidence underscores the physiological basis of empathy and rapport. Mirror neurons activate during empathic engagement, facilitating attunement between clinician and patient. Consistent, respectful dialogue modulates the patient's autonomic arousal, promoting calm and trust. This neurobiological dimension of therapeutic presence validates the PMHNP's role in emotional regulation during sessions.

Therapeutic boundaries preserve professional integrity and patient safety. Overidentification or emotional entanglement compromises objectivity. The practitioner maintains empathy without assumption, authenticity without overdisclosure. Regular supervision and reflective journaling help monitor countertransference—those personal reactions that can unconsciously influence clinical judgment.

Trauma-Informed Care

Trauma-informed care recognizes the pervasive impact of trauma on mental and physical health. The PMHNP approaches all interactions with an assumption of potential trauma exposure. Core principles include safety, trustworthiness, choice, collaboration, and empowerment. These values guide tone of voice, physical environment, and pacing of assessment.

Physiologically, trauma imprints on the limbic system, heightening reactivity and altering cortisol regulation. Clinicians who overlook trauma risk retraumatization through abrupt questioning or invasive procedures. Instead, the PMHNP establishes predictability, explains each step, and seeks consent continuously.

Interventions integrate grounding techniques, mindfulness, and stabilization before exploration of traumatic memories. Collaboration with therapists trained in Eye Movement Desensitization and Reprocessing (EMDR) or somatic therapies ensures continuity of trauma recovery. The PMHNP's role includes pharmacologic management of hyperarousal and sleep disturbance, education about neurobiological responses, and validation of resilience rather than pathology.

Trauma-informed systems extend beyond individual practice to institutional culture. Policies supporting staff wellness, debriefing after crises, and transparent communication embody the same principles offered to patients, promoting collective resilience in healthcare teams.

Cultural and Spiritual Competence

Cultural competence transforms awareness into practice. The PMHNP interprets behaviors, expressions of distress, and health beliefs through the lens of each patient's cultural context. Language barriers, migration experiences, and differing explanatory models of illness influence engagement and adherence.

Cultural humility surpasses technical competence. It requires ongoing self-evaluation, acknowledgment of bias, and openness to learning from the patient. Instead of assuming expertise, the clinician invites narratives: "Can you tell me what you believe is happening?" Such inquiry fosters respect and uncovers metaphors that align biomedical treatment with personal meaning.

Spiritual assessment complements cultural inquiry. For many patients, spirituality provides coping structure, community, and moral guidance. The PMHNP may use frameworks like **FICA** (Faith, Importance, Community, Address) to integrate spiritual dimensions ethically. Collaboration with chaplains or faith leaders occurs only with consent. Recognizing the interface between spiritual crisis and psychiatric symptoms—such as differentiating mystical experience from psychosis—requires clinical sensitivity and nonjudgmental curiosity.

Interprofessional Collaboration and Systems-Based Practice

Psychiatric care operates within a multidisciplinary framework. The PMHNP collaborates with psychiatrists, psychologists, primary care providers, social workers, and occupational therapists to deliver coordinated, patient-centered care. Each discipline contributes unique expertise: psychiatrists provide diagnostic and pharmacologic oversight; psychologists offer psychotherapeutic specialization; social workers navigate community resources.

Effective collaboration relies on mutual respect and clarity of role boundaries. The PMHNP functions as a bridge between medical and psychosocial models, translating complex neurobiological findings into accessible explanations for team members and patients. Regular case conferences and documentation in shared electronic health records promote transparency and continuity.

Systems-based practice also encompasses understanding healthcare economics, policy, and quality improvement. Nurse practitioners advocate for equitable access to mental health services, addressing disparities rooted in socioeconomic and geographic inequities. By participating in program development and policy committees, PMHNPs extend influence beyond individual encounters to systemic transformation.

Documentation, Informatics, and Legal Safeguards

Documentation serves as both a clinical record and a legal instrument. The PMHNP records assessments, diagnoses, treatment plans, and patient responses in a manner that is accurate, objective, and timely. Language must reflect observation rather than interpretation—for example, "patient paced the floor for ten minutes" rather than "patient appeared agitated."

Electronic health records (EHRs) require proficiency in privacy standards under HIPAA and related state laws. The practitioner safeguards patient data, employs secure communication channels, and exercises caution when sharing information across systems. Documentation should include rationale for clinical decisions, informed consent discussions, and evidence of patient education.

In legal proceedings, records serve as testimony of care quality. Thorough documentation demonstrates adherence to professional standards and ethical duty. The PMHNP remains aware that every entry may be reviewed by peers, auditors, or legal entities, reinforcing the necessity for precision and professionalism.

Clinical Leadership and Quality Improvement

Leadership within advanced practice nursing extends beyond supervision. The PMHNP exemplifies clinical excellence, mentors peers, and contributes to the culture of safety. Leadership is exercised through role modeling, ethical decision-making, and advocacy for evidence-based practice.

Quality improvement (QI) initiatives rely on systematic evaluation of outcomes. The PMHNP participates in root cause analyses after sentinel events, designs protocols to reduce medication errors, and implements patient feedback mechanisms. Familiarity with models such as Plan–Do–Study–Act (PDSA) cycles supports iterative refinement of care processes.

In mental health settings, leadership also includes emotional intelligence—the capacity to regulate one's own emotions and inspire resilience in others. Leaders foster environments where staff feel valued, reducing burnout and turnover. Through scholarly dissemination and continuing education, PMHNPs advance the profession's collective knowledge base.

Ethical Communication and Professional Boundaries in Practice

Every clinical interaction carries ethical implications. The PMHNP navigates confidentiality, informed consent, and professional power dynamics while maintaining therapeutic effectiveness. Patients may disclose sensitive information, develop dependency, or test boundaries. The practitioner balances empathy with firmness, maintaining a professional stance grounded in respect and transparency.

When ethical uncertainty arises, consultation with colleagues or institutional ethics committees supports sound decision-making. For instance, when a patient refuses medication despite risk of relapse, the PMHNP weighs autonomy against beneficence, seeking least-restrictive alternatives. Documentation of deliberation and consultation demonstrates accountability.

Boundary integrity extends to digital communication. Social media, email, and telehealth introduce new ethical landscapes. The PMHNP avoids dual relationships and ensures virtual platforms meet confidentiality standards. Ethical practice sustains trust—the cornerstone of advanced psychiatric nursing.

Integrative View of Advanced Practice Competency

Domain II culminates in synthesis: technical skill, interpersonal acuity, and ethical mindfulness unite to define advanced practice excellence. The PMHNP operates simultaneously as scientist, clinician, advocate, and leader. Every assessment, conversation, and intervention reflects a deep understanding of human complexity and system responsibility.

Mastery of advanced skills does not rest solely on knowledge acquisition but on reflection-in-action—the capacity to adapt theory to the unpredictable dynamics of human experience. The PMHNP's ongoing self-awareness, cultural curiosity, and commitment to evidence-based innovation transform clinical encounters into opportunities for healing and growth.

Through disciplined practice and compassionate insight, the advanced psychiatric nurse practitioner fulfills the profession's highest mandate: to promote holistic mental health with integrity, competence, and humanity.

Scan QR Code to get Flashcards and Audio File

Chapter 3: Diagnosis and Treatment

Accurate diagnosis is the cornerstone of effective psychiatric care. The PMHNP synthesizes data from interviews, physical assessments, psychological testing, and collateral reports to determine the nature of a disorder. Diagnosis according to the DSM-5-TR provides a standardized language for clinical communication but must always be interpreted within individual context.

Understanding the DSM-5-TR Framework

The DSM-5-TR categorizes mental disorders based on symptom clusters, duration, and functional impairment. It represents a descriptive taxonomy rather than a theory of etiology. The PMHNP interprets these classifications with clinical discernment, considering comorbidities and overlapping presentations. For example, anxiety may manifest within mood disorders, and psychosis can arise in both schizophrenia and severe depression.

The diagnostic process proceeds through systematic steps: identifying the chief complaint, obtaining a psychiatric and medical history, assessing current symptoms, and ruling out physiological or substance-related causes. Cultural and developmental factors shape symptom expression; thus, the practitioner integrates cultural formulation interviews when appropriate.

Differential diagnosis requires attention to temporal patterns. Transient stress reactions differ from persistent disorders; substance-induced mood disturbances resolve upon detoxification, distinguishing them from primary mood disorders. Each diagnosis entails verification through objective findings and clinical reasoning rather than checklist adherence.

Evidence-Based Treatment Planning

Once diagnosis is established, treatment planning aligns evidence-based interventions with patient preferences and available resources. The PMHNP evaluates clinical guidelines, research evidence, and real-world feasibility. Collaboration with patients ensures adherence and autonomy.

For depressive disorders, evidence supports combined pharmacotherapy and cognitive-behavioral therapy as superior to either alone. Anxiety disorders respond to exposure-based therapies with or without medication. Psychotic disorders require antipsychotic therapy integrated with psychosocial rehabilitation.

Treatment planning includes measurable goals, time frames, and evaluation criteria. The PMHNP continually reassesses progress, adjusting modalities as symptoms evolve. Interprofessional communication—particularly with psychiatrists, psychologists, and primary care providers—enhances continuity of care and safety.

Complementary and Alternative Treatments

Beyond conventional medicine, complementary approaches expand patient choice. Mindfulness-based stress reduction, yoga, and nutritional supplementation have gained empirical support for mood regulation. The PMHNP evaluates evidence quality, potential interactions, and patient expectations. For instance, St. John's Wort may alleviate mild depression but interacts with SSRIs, risking serotonin syndrome.

Cultural humility remains essential when patients employ traditional remedies. The practitioner validates belief systems while ensuring safety through education and monitoring. Integrative care requires balance—respecting diversity without compromising evidence-based standards.

Psychopharmacotherapeutic Management

Psychopharmacology represents both art and science. The PMHNP applies knowledge of receptor dynamics, neural circuitry, and patient individuality to select and titrate medications safely. Every decision integrates symptom pattern, medical comorbidity, previous drug response, and patient preference.

Antidepressants remain central to treatment of mood disorders. Selective serotonin reuptake inhibitors (SSRIs) such as sertraline and escitalopram provide favorable tolerability, whereas serotonin–norepinephrine reuptake inhibitors (SNRIs) address concomitant pain or fatigue. The nurse practitioner evaluates onset latency, typically four to six weeks, and monitors for early agitation or gastrointestinal upset. In partial response, dosage adjustment precedes augmentation with atypical agents or psychotherapy.

Mood stabilizers—lithium, valproate, carbamazepine, and lamotrigine—require serum level monitoring to prevent toxicity. Lithium's neuroprotective effects make it unique in suicide prevention, yet renal and thyroid surveillance are mandatory. The PMHNP counsels regarding hydration, consistent salt intake, and early signs of toxicity such as tremor or ataxia.

Antipsychotics divide into first- and second-generation classes. Second-generation agents (e.g., risperidone, quetiapine, aripiprazole) combine dopamine D2 and serotonin 5-HT2A antagonism, improving negative symptoms and reducing extrapyramidal side effects. Metabolic monitoring—weight, waist circumference, glucose, and lipids—protects against long-term complications.

Anxiolytics include benzodiazepines for short-term relief and non-benzodiazepine options such as buspirone, hydroxyzine, or certain antidepressants for chronic anxiety. Caution is essential to avoid dependence. The PMHNP employs tapering schedules and cognitive-behavioral support when discontinuing sedatives.

Stimulants and non-stimulants treat attention-deficit/hyperactivity disorder across the lifespan. Monitoring of blood pressure, appetite, and sleep is integral. Comorbid mood or substance-use disorders necessitate modified protocols emphasizing behavioral structure and psychosocial therapy.

Pharmacologic Decision-Making and Polypharmacy

The complexity of psychiatric illness often leads to polypharmacy—use of multiple medications simultaneously. The PMHNP exercises restraint and scientific reasoning, adding agents only with clear rationale. Each addition must address a defined target symptom, demonstrate benefit, and minimize interaction risk.

Pharmacokinetic considerations guide scheduling and dosage: hepatic enzyme induction, protein binding, and renal clearance vary across drugs and individuals. Polypharmacy increases potential for adverse effects, adherence challenges, and financial burden. Simplification through cross-tapering or combination products enhances safety and compliance.

Evidence synthesis informs practice. The PMHNP consults systematic reviews, meta-analyses, and national guidelines to justify treatment combinations. Ongoing outcome tracking ensures accountability.

Non-Pharmacologic and Integrative Interventions

Medication alone rarely achieves full recovery. The PMHNP incorporates psychotherapeutic, behavioral, and somatic modalities tailored to diagnosis and patient readiness.

Cognitive-behavioral therapy (CBT) restructures maladaptive thinking and behaviors; dialectical behavior therapy (DBT) stabilizes emotion in borderline personality disorder; interpersonal therapy (IPT) focuses on role transitions and grief. Understanding theoretical foundations allows the PMHNP to reinforce therapeutic principles during routine visits, creating a seamless blend of pharmacologic and psychologic care.

Somatic treatments such as electroconvulsive therapy (ECT), repetitive transcranial magnetic stimulation (rTMS), and emerging neuromodulation techniques remain options for treatment-resistant conditions. The nurse practitioner educates patients about indications, mechanisms, and side-effect profiles, coordinating with psychiatrists for procedural oversight.

Lifestyle interventions—sleep hygiene, physical activity, and balanced nutrition—carry robust evidence for symptom improvement. Exercise enhances neurogenesis and endorphin release, while structured sleep restores circadian alignment. The PMHNP's role includes motivational coaching and accountability within holistic care plans.

Diagnostic Reasoning and Clinical Formulation

Diagnostic reasoning combines inductive and deductive thinking. The PMHNP gathers data, identifies salient features, hypothesizes explanations, and tests them against evidence. Clinical formulation synthesizes biological, psychological, and social dimensions into a coherent narrative that guides treatment.

Key elements include:

Predisposing factors such as genetics or early trauma.
Precipitating events like loss or substance use.
Perpetuating influences including maladaptive coping or environment.
Protective resources such as support networks or faith.
Formulation translates beyond labeling—it explains how symptoms developed and persist. By articulating mechanisms, the PMHNP designs interventions targeting underlying processes rather than surface manifestations.

Comorbidity and Differential Diagnosis

Psychiatric and medical comorbidities intertwine. Depression co-occurs with cardiovascular disease, diabetes, and chronic pain; anxiety amplifies asthma and gastrointestinal disorders. Substance use frequently masks or mimics primary mental illness.

The PMHNP evaluates cross-system symptoms to avoid misattribution. Laboratory tests—thyroid function, B12, folate, electrolytes—exclude metabolic causes. Neurologic evaluation rules out seizure or movement disorders presenting as psychiatric disturbance.

Differential diagnosis demands awareness of medication side effects: corticosteroids may induce mania, beta-blockers provoke depression, and stimulants can trigger anxiety. By integrating medical review and psychiatric assessment, the practitioner ensures holistic accuracy.

Measurement-Based Care and Outcome Evaluation

Measurement-based care (MBC) transforms subjective observation into quantifiable progress tracking. The PMHNP implements standardized scales—PHQ-9, GAD-7, Brief Psychiatric Rating Scale, or Young Mania Rating Scale—at baseline and regular intervals.

Data inform decisions: a 50 percent reduction in PHQ-9 indicates clinical response; persistent elevation triggers treatment adjustment. MBC enhances patient engagement, as visible metrics validate improvement. It also satisfies quality-assurance standards demanded by payers and accreditation bodies.

Documentation of outcomes fosters accountability and research literacy. The PMHNP interprets change scores alongside narrative assessment, ensuring numbers complement rather than replace human understanding.

Treatment Adherence and Therapeutic Alliance

Adherence emerges from alliance, not instruction. The PMHNP explores barriers—side effects, cost, stigma, misunderstanding—and negotiates solutions collaboratively. Shared decision-making empowers patients, improving retention and outcomes.

Motivational strategies reinforce autonomy: "What benefits have you noticed?" or "What concerns do you still have?" Such dialogue transforms compliance into partnership. Adherence education includes written instructions, follow-up reminders, and crisis access information.

Therapeutic alliance extends to families and caregivers when appropriate. Their inclusion fosters continuity, particularly for those with severe or chronic illness. Trust and respect remain the strongest predictors of adherence and recovery.

Long-Term Management and Relapse Prevention

Chronic psychiatric disorders require maintenance beyond acute stabilization. The PMHNP establishes long-term follow-up intervals, monitoring medication levels, metabolic health, and psychosocial functioning. Relapse prevention includes early warning sign identification and crisis planning.

Psychoeducation equips patients to self-monitor: sleep disruption, irritability, or social withdrawal often precede recurrence. Prompt adjustment of therapy or dosage prevents full relapse. Integration with community resources—support groups, vocational programs, peer specialists—sustains recovery in real-world settings.

Continuity of care embodies ethical responsibility. Through consistent presence, documentation, and advocacy, the PMHNP ensures that healing becomes sustainable, not episodic.

Disorder-Specific Pharmacologic Strategies

Mood Disorders

The PMHNP differentiates unipolar from bipolar depression to avoid iatrogenic destabilization. Antidepressant monotherapy in bipolar depression can precipitate mania; therefore, mood stabilizers or atypical antipsychotics form first-line therapy. For unipolar depression, SSRIs or SNRIs remain the mainstay, with augmentation using atypical agents or psychotherapy for partial responders.

Treatment-resistant depression demands systematic evaluation—confirming adherence, diagnosis accuracy, and medical contributors. Options include switching classes, combining agents (e.g., SSRI plus bupropion), or introducing somatic therapies such as transcranial magnetic stimulation. The PMHNP evaluates for emerging interventions, including ketamine and esketamine nasal formulations, which modulate glutamate pathways to produce rapid antidepressant effects.

Anxiety and Trauma-Related Disorders

Anxiety management integrates pharmacologic stabilization and cognitive-behavioral restructuring. SSRIs and SNRIs serve as first-line agents, while benzodiazepines offer short-term relief during acute crises. The practitioner vigilantly monitors for dependence, tapering gradually when anxiety is controlled.

Post-traumatic stress disorder (PTSD) requires trauma-informed pharmacotherapy—targeting hyperarousal and intrusive re-experiencing. Sertraline and paroxetine have FDA approval; prazosin reduces nightmares by blocking central adrenergic activation. Psychotherapy remains integral, but medication provides physiological calm that enables cognitive processing.

Psychotic Disorders

Schizophrenia and schizoaffective disorders demand lifelong, individualized management. Second-generation antipsychotics balance efficacy and metabolic risk. Clozapine remains superior for treatment-resistant psychosis but mandates hematologic monitoring. The PMHNP coordinates regular complete blood counts and educates patients on early signs of agranulocytosis or myocarditis.

Long-acting injectable formulations (LAIs) enhance adherence and reduce relapse. The practitioner assesses patient readiness and provides education regarding administration schedules. Integration with psychosocial rehabilitation—skills training, supported employment, and family education—optimizes functional outcomes.

Substance Use and Co-Occurring Disorders

Co-occurring disorders require concurrent, not sequential, treatment. The PMHNP employs motivational interviewing to strengthen readiness and pharmacotherapies such as buprenorphine, methadone, or naltrexone for opioid dependence; acamprosate or disulfiram for alcohol use disorder.

Psychotropic selection considers hepatic metabolism and risk of interaction. Antidepressants like sertraline and mirtazapine can be safely used during recovery, while bupropion aids smoking cessation when seizure risk is low. Collaboration with addiction specialists and community programs ensures comprehensive rehabilitation.

Crisis Stabilization and Acute Care Management

Acute psychiatric crises—suicidal ideation, violent behavior, or psychotic disorganization—test both clinical acumen and emotional resilience. The PMHNP's immediate objective is safety through rapid assessment, environmental control, and pharmacologic intervention when needed.

In acute mania, high-dose atypical antipsychotics and benzodiazepines reduce agitation before introducing mood stabilizers. For acute psychosis, intramuscular haloperidol with lorazepam remains a standard emergency combination when oral therapy is refused.

Suicidal crises demand structured evaluation of intent, means, and protective factors. Hospitalization or involuntary hold may be necessary under duty-to-protect statutes. Crisis stabilization involves not only medication but also emotional containment—calm voice, presence, and reassurance of care continuity. After stabilization, follow-up within one week is critical to maintain engagement and adjust therapy.

Children and Adolescents

Pediatric psychiatric care emphasizes developmental context and family involvement. The PMHNP conducts age-appropriate interviews using play or creative activities. Pharmacologic treatment begins with minimal effective dosages, titrated cautiously. SSRIs (fluoxetine, escitalopram) are approved for pediatric depression; stimulants and non-stimulants address ADHD. Monitoring includes growth, appetite, and suicidality due to heightened vulnerability during initiation.

Family psychoeducation is essential to address misconceptions, encourage adherence, and set realistic expectations. Collaboration with schools ensures academic support and early detection of behavioral shifts.

Perinatal Mental Health

During pregnancy and postpartum, the PMHNP balances maternal well-being and fetal safety. Untreated depression carries obstetric and developmental risks, whereas certain medications pose teratogenic potential. SSRIs such as sertraline have the most favorable safety profile; paroxetine and valproate are avoided.

Postpartum depression and psychosis require urgent recognition. Lactation considerations influence drug choice, as many psychotropics are excreted in breast milk. The practitioner collaborates with obstetricians, pediatricians, and lactation consultants to individualize care.

Geriatric Psychiatry

Older adults present unique pharmacokinetic vulnerabilities: reduced renal clearance, polypharmacy, and cognitive decline increase risk of adverse effects. The PMHNP starts with "low and slow" dosing, prioritizing safety. SSRIs (except paroxetine) are preferred for depression; antipsychotics carry black-box warnings in dementia-related psychosis and must be justified carefully.

Cognitive assessment distinguishes depression-induced pseudodementia from true neurocognitive disorders. Nonpharmacologic interventions—structured routine, reminiscence therapy, social engagement—enhance cognitive reserve and quality of life.

Culturally Responsive Diagnosis and Treatment

Cultural context shapes symptom expression, help-seeking behavior, and therapeutic alliance. The PMHNP employs the **Cultural Formulation Interview** to explore patient identity, explanatory models, stressors, and support systems. Recognizing idioms of distress prevents misdiagnosis—for example, somatic presentations of depression in some cultures or spiritual framing of hallucinations in others.

Treatment planning integrates cultural beliefs with biomedical approaches. The practitioner respects traditional healers or community rituals when safe, building trust through humility and shared decision-making. Language interpreters facilitate accuracy, but emotional tone and nonverbal respect remain equally vital.

Cultural competence is dynamic; ongoing reflection, supervision, and community engagement sustain authenticity. By honoring cultural diversity, the PMHNP strengthens adherence and equity in mental health outcomes.

Emerging and Innovative Treatments

Psychiatric nursing evolves alongside neuroscience. The PMHNP stays informed about innovative modalities:

Ketamine and Esketamine for treatment-resistant depression—rapid action through NMDA receptor modulation.

Psychedelic-assisted therapy (under clinical investigation) exploring psilocybin's role in existential distress and PTSD.
Digital therapeutics delivering cognitive-behavioral interventions via mobile platforms.
Neurofeedback training brainwave regulation for attention and anxiety disorders.
While promising, these innovations require critical appraisal of safety, ethics, and evidence quality. The PMHNP educates patients honestly, distinguishing emerging research from established practice. Integrating innovation responsibly ensures advancement without compromising standards.

Integrating Case Reasoning: A Clinical Example

A 42-year-old patient presents with low mood, insomnia, and poor concentration. The PMHNP conducts thorough assessment, ruling out thyroid dysfunction and substance use. History reveals childhood trauma and family depression. Diagnosis: Major depressive disorder, recurrent, moderate.

Treatment begins with sertraline, psychoeducation on neurobiology of depression, and cognitive-behavioral therapy referral. After four weeks, partial improvement prompts dose increase. Measurement-based tracking shows PHQ-9 reduction from 18 to 9. Patient gains energy, resumes exercise, and reports renewed motivation.

This case exemplifies integrated reasoning—biological, psychological, and social domains combined through evidence-based intervention, empathic engagement, and outcome evaluation.

Ethical Dimensions of Treatment Decisions

Ethical challenges permeate clinical decision-making. Balancing beneficence, autonomy, and justice requires nuanced judgment. The PMHNP ensures informed consent for every pharmacologic and psychotherapeutic decision, discusses risks transparently, and respects patient refusal unless imminent danger exists.

Medication coercion, resource limitation, and cultural conflict demand reflection and consultation. Ethical documentation of reasoning protects both patient and practitioner. By modeling ethical integrity, the PMHNP fosters trust essential to long-term healing.

Integrated Treatment Systems and Continuum of Care

Modern psychiatric care operates within a continuum that spans acute stabilization to community reintegration. The PMHNP serves as both clinician and care coordinator, ensuring continuity across inpatient, outpatient, and community settings. Fragmentation of care contributes to relapse and nonadherence; therefore, communication among providers and consistent follow-up are paramount.

Integrated treatment models unite behavioral health with primary care. Collaborative care frameworks embed mental health practitioners within medical teams, using shared records and structured outcome monitoring. Evidence demonstrates improved depression remission and reduced hospitalization rates when collaborative protocols are implemented. The PMHNP leads or participates in these systems, interpreting data, advising on psychopharmacology, and mentoring primary care staff on psychiatric screening and referral.

Transitions between levels of care require meticulous handoffs. Discharge planning includes medication reconciliation, crisis contacts, and scheduled appointments within seven days of hospital release. The PMHNP reinforces education about early relapse indicators, fosters self-management skills, and connects patients with peer or community supports.

Chronic Disease Management and Longitudinal Care

Chronic psychiatric conditions mirror other long-term illnesses such as diabetes or hypertension—requiring ongoing monitoring and lifestyle adaptation. The PMHNP establishes longitudinal relationships, cultivating trust and continuity. Regular follow-up evaluates not only symptoms but functional recovery: employment, relationships, self-care, and community engagement.

Collaborative goal setting enhances empowerment. Patients define personal recovery milestones—returning to work, reestablishing social ties, pursuing education—and the PMHNP structures care around these outcomes. Chronic care management includes medication adherence, metabolic monitoring, and comorbidity screening for cardiovascular or endocrine disorders associated with psychotropic use.

Integration of motivational interviewing supports behavior change and health literacy. Patients learn to interpret their mood charts, medication schedules, and side-effect patterns. This active participation strengthens autonomy, reduces crisis episodes, and improves quality of life.

Relapse Prevention Frameworks

Relapse prevention is a dynamic process rooted in awareness, anticipation, and resilience. The PMHNP educates patients to identify personal triggers—stress, substance use, sleep disruption—and develop proactive coping strategies. Relapse is reframed not as failure but as an opportunity for recalibration.

In mood disorders, early warning signs include irritability, sleep reduction, and impulsive spending; in psychotic disorders, subtle changes in speech or social withdrawal often precede decompensation. Collaborative monitoring tools such as daily mood logs or mobile health apps provide early alerts.

Pharmacologic maintenance—such as lithium or depot antipsychotics—reduces recurrence, but psychosocial factors sustain stability. Support networks, vocational engagement, and meaningful activity maintain momentum. The PMHNP ensures multidisciplinary coordination so that therapy, medication, and community resources function as a cohesive safety net.

Outcome Evaluation and Quality Metrics

Outcome evaluation quantifies treatment effectiveness and guides quality improvement. The PMHNP employs multiple metrics: symptom scales, functional indices, patient satisfaction, and biological markers such as weight or glucose. Data collection aligns with quality frameworks like the **National Committee for Quality Assurance (NCQA)** behavioral health standards.

Statistical literacy allows the practitioner to interpret effect sizes, confidence intervals, and clinical significance. Improvement is judged not only by score reduction but by restoration of life roles. Continuous performance monitoring ensures accountability and informs program development.

Quality metrics extend beyond individual care to organizational performance—reducing readmissions, improving adherence rates, and closing disparities in minority populations. PMHNPs contribute by analyzing aggregate data, proposing evidence-based interventions, and leading implementation teams.

Telepsychiatry and Digital Integration

Telepsychiatry has redefined accessibility in mental healthcare. The PMHNP uses secure video platforms to reach patients in remote or underserved regions. Success depends on maintaining therapeutic presence despite physical distance. Eye contact, tone modulation, and empathetic pacing compensate for reduced sensory cues.

Telehealth requires compliance with privacy regulations, licensure reciprocity, and informed consent adapted to virtual contexts. Documentation specifies platform security, patient location, and emergency protocol.

Digital tools extend beyond live video. Remote monitoring apps track mood and medication adherence; secure messaging provides timely check-ins. These technologies enhance engagement and allow early intervention. Yet boundaries remain crucial—communication outside scheduled sessions must preserve professionalism and confidentiality.

The PMHNP integrates technology judiciously, combining innovation with human connection. Technology supports, but never replaces, the therapeutic relationship.

Leadership in Evidence-Based Practice

Evidence-based practice (EBP) anchors modern psychiatric nursing in scientific rigor. The PMHNP critically appraises research, integrates clinical expertise, and honors patient values. Implementing EBP involves framing clinical questions using the **PICO** model (Population, Intervention, Comparison, Outcome), searching literature systematically, and translating findings into actionable protocols.

Leadership emerges through mentorship and advocacy. The PMHNP guides teams in adopting clinical pathways, contributes to policy committees, and promotes continuing education. Translational scholarship—bridging research and bedside care—ensures that evidence informs daily decisions.

Barriers to EBP include resource limitations, resistance to change, and data overload. Skilled leaders foster a culture of inquiry, encouraging staff to question tradition and pursue improvement. Through journal clubs, case conferences, and QI projects, PMHNPs transform evidence into sustainable practice.

Ethics and Patient-Centered Outcomes

The essence of diagnosis and treatment lies in honoring autonomy and dignity. Ethical reasoning accompanies every prescription and care plan. Informed consent is ongoing, not a one-time signature. The PMHNP ensures comprehension, accommodates literacy levels, and invites questions.

Patient-centered outcomes redefine success beyond symptom remission. Recovery means agency, self-acceptance, and life participation. The practitioner measures progress in satisfaction, social contribution, and resilience. Ethical fidelity demands responsiveness to each person's evolving goals rather than rigid adherence to clinical algorithms.

The advanced PMHNP thus blends science with empathy, analytics with artistry. Diagnosis and treatment culminate not merely in stability but in empowerment—a restoration of personhood within the complexity of modern healthcare.

Chapter 4: Psychotherapy and Related Theories

The Role of Psychotherapy in Advanced Psychiatric Nursing

Psychotherapy is a core competency of the psychiatric–mental health nurse practitioner. It reflects the synthesis of scientific knowledge, interpersonal skill, and ethical awareness. The PMHNP applies psychotherapeutic principles to promote emotional growth, behavioral change, and resilience across the lifespan.

While medication addresses biological symptoms, psychotherapy modifies cognitive and relational patterns that sustain distress. The therapeutic relationship itself functions as an agent of change—an environment where patients experience acceptance, understanding, and empowerment.

Psychotherapy demands disciplined self-awareness. The PMHNP uses introspection to recognize countertransference, biases, and emotional resonance. By observing one's own reactions, the practitioner refines empathy into precision. The process transforms both patient and clinician, affirming the humanistic foundation of psychiatric care.

Major Theoretical Frameworks

Psychotherapy derives from multiple schools of thought. Though distinct in technique, all share the goal of fostering self-understanding and adaptive functioning. The PMHNP must grasp each theory's conceptual model, mechanism of change, and clinical indications.

1. Psychodynamic Theory

Rooted in Freud's early work and refined by modern object-relations and self-psychology theorists, psychodynamic therapy explores unconscious processes shaping emotion and behavior. Key concepts include transference, defense mechanisms, and early attachment patterns.

The PMHNP employing psychodynamic principles listens for recurrent themes, symbolic meanings, and emotional undercurrents. Insight emerges when unconscious conflicts become conscious, enabling choice rather than compulsion. Modern brief psychodynamic therapy adapts this depth model to structured, time-limited care.

2. Cognitive-Behavioral Theory

Cognitive-behavioral therapy (CBT) asserts that thoughts influence emotions and behavior. Dysfunction arises from distorted cognition—catastrophizing, overgeneralization, or all-or-nothing thinking. Through structured sessions, patients identify and reframe maladaptive thoughts, practice behavioral experiments, and build coping strategies.

The PMHNP integrates CBT techniques even within medication visits: challenging negative self-talk, assigning behavioral activation tasks, or using thought records. Evidence supports CBT for depression, anxiety, insomnia, and chronic pain. Its collaborative, measurable nature aligns well with outcome-oriented nursing practice.

3. Humanistic and Existential Theories

Humanistic approaches emphasize authenticity, empathy, and unconditional positive regard. Existential therapy expands this stance into philosophical exploration of meaning, freedom, and responsibility. The

PMHNP helps patients confront existential anxieties—death, isolation, and choice—while discovering purpose and agency.

This approach suits patients seeking personal growth beyond symptom relief. Techniques include empathic reflection, here-and-now awareness, and exploration of values. The therapeutic stance is nonjudgmental and genuine, allowing healing through relational authenticity.

4. Behavioral and Learning Theories

Behavioral therapy applies principles of conditioning to modify observable actions. Techniques such as exposure, systematic desensitization, and operant reinforcement reshape maladaptive responses. For example, graded exposure diminishes phobic avoidance by pairing anxiety triggers with relaxation until fear extinguishes.

The PMHNP integrates behavioral strategies in anxiety, trauma, and substance-use care, encouraging measurable skill development. Behavioral activation—engaging in positive activities despite low motivation—has proven especially effective in depression management.

5. Family Systems Theory

Family systems therapy views the individual within the relational network. Symptoms often represent dysfunction in communication, boundaries, or roles. The PMHNP assesses patterns such as triangulation, enmeshment, or rigid hierarchies.

Intervention focuses on altering interaction sequences rather than blaming members. Genograms map generational patterns; reframing promotes understanding instead of conflict. Systems thinking enriches the PMHNP's holistic approach, recognizing that individual healing reverberates through the family unit.

6. Feminist and Multicultural Theories

Feminist and multicultural frameworks situate psychological distress within sociocultural power structures. They emphasize equality, empowerment, and social justice. The PMHNP practicing from this lens validates the impact of discrimination, gender roles, and cultural expectations on mental health.

Therapeutic dialogue invites reflection on identity, privilege, and resilience. The goal is collaborative, not hierarchical: clinician and client co-create understanding. These models resonate strongly with nursing's ethical principles of advocacy and respect for human dignity.

Integrative and Eclectic Approaches

Few practitioners adhere rigidly to one theory. The PMHNP blends models according to patient needs—a process known as theoretical integration. Cognitive-behavioral skills may combine with mindfulness, psychodynamic insight, or family interventions.

Integrative therapy requires coherence rather than eclecticism. The clinician articulates a unifying rationale linking chosen methods to presenting problems. Evidence-based integration ensures that techniques are applied intentionally rather than arbitrarily.

Case formulation guides this synthesis. For a patient with trauma-related depression, treatment may begin with grounding and CBT for safety, followed by psychodynamic exploration of attachment wounds once stability is achieved. Flexibility allows adaptation without sacrificing structure.

The Therapeutic Relationship

Regardless of modality, the therapeutic relationship is the primary vehicle of change. Trust, empathy, congruence, and respect establish the alliance. Research consistently identifies therapeutic alliance as the strongest predictor of outcome, surpassing specific technique.

The PMHNP cultivates presence—attentive silence, responsive listening, and acceptance. Boundaries create safety; authenticity invites honesty. Repairing ruptures—acknowledging misunderstandings or emotional missteps—strengthens trust and models healthy communication.

Transference and countertransference offer valuable data. When a patient idealizes, resists, or challenges the clinician, underlying relational templates surface. The PMHNP responds with curiosity and professionalism, using these dynamics to illuminate patterns rather than react personally.

Therapeutic Process and Phases

Psychotherapy unfolds in phases: engagement, exploration, working, and termination. Each stage demands different clinician tasks.

Engagement Phase: Establish rapport, clarify goals, and create safety. The PMHNP explains confidentiality and session structure. Early success builds motivation.
Exploration Phase: Patient narratives deepen. The practitioner listens for themes, validates emotions, and identifies maladaptive beliefs. Insight and alliance expand.
Working Phase: Active change occurs—challenging cognitions, experimenting with behaviors, or confronting avoided emotions. Resistance is expected and explored.
Termination Phase: Gains are consolidated. The PMHNP reviews progress, reinforces skills, and discusses relapse prevention. Termination symbolizes mastery and autonomy.
Ending therapy evokes mixed emotions; open discussion honors the therapeutic journey and models healthy closure.

Mindfulness and Third-Wave Therapies

Third-wave behavioral therapies incorporate acceptance, mindfulness, and contextual awareness. **Acceptance and Commitment Therapy (ACT)** teaches psychological flexibility—observing thoughts without judgment while committing to value-driven action. **Dialectical Behavior Therapy (DBT)** integrates mindfulness with emotion regulation and interpersonal effectiveness, particularly effective for borderline personality disorder.

The PMHNP integrates mindfulness exercises—breath awareness, body scanning, and grounding—into daily practice. These interventions reduce rumination, improve distress tolerance, and complement pharmacologic management. Mindfulness-based cognitive therapy has demonstrated efficacy in preventing depressive relapse by strengthening metacognitive awareness.

Group Psychotherapy

Group therapy offers unique therapeutic mechanisms: universality, shared identification, altruism, and interpersonal learning. Under skilled facilitation, members provide feedback, test new behaviors, and gain perspective on relational patterns.

The PMHNP designs groups around specific themes—depression management, trauma recovery, medication adherence, or coping with chronic illness. Group norms emphasize confidentiality, respect, and participation. The leader balances process (emotional interaction) and content (topic discussion).

Group dynamics reveal transference phenomena within the collective; the PMHNP intervenes to maintain safety and cohesion. Group therapy's cost-effectiveness and mutual support align with community-based mental health priorities.

Evidence-Based Psychotherapy Integration

Empirical support guides therapeutic selection. Meta-analyses consistently affirm CBT, interpersonal therapy, and behavioral activation for depression; exposure-based therapies for anxiety; DBT for borderline personality disorder; and family interventions for schizophrenia.

The PMHNP evaluates evidence strength, considers cultural relevance, and matches interventions to patient readiness. Fidelity to evidence-based methods ensures accountability, while individualized adaptation honors person-centered care.

Supervision and continuing education sustain competence. The clinician engages in peer consultation, outcome monitoring, and self-reflection to refine skill and prevent drift from established protocols.

Supervision, Reflective Practice, and Therapist Growth

Ongoing supervision safeguards quality and nurtures professional growth. Through reflective dialogue, the PMHNP explores emotional responses, ethical dilemmas, and theoretical uncertainties. Supervision transforms experience into wisdom, reducing burnout and enhancing empathy.

Reflective practice extends beyond formal supervision. Journaling, mindfulness, and self-assessment cultivate self-awareness. Recognition of personal limitations and bias preserves therapeutic neutrality. The effective therapist remains a lifelong learner, blending humility with confidence.

Cultural and Ethical Dimensions in Psychotherapy

Cultural awareness within therapy transcends language—it encompasses worldview, family norms, and expressions of emotion. The PMHNP avoids pathologizing culturally normative behaviors, demonstrating curiosity and respect.

Ethical practice ensures confidentiality, informed consent, and clear boundaries. Dual relationships and role conflicts are avoided. The PMHNP documents consent processes, progress notes, and supervision encounters meticulously. Ethics also involves advocacy—challenging systemic inequities affecting mental health access and treatment.

Psychotherapy rooted in ethics and culture upholds nursing's moral mission: to affirm humanity and justice in every therapeutic encounter.

Psychotherapy as a discipline is both art and science. It calls for intellectual rigor balanced by emotional sensitivity. In advanced psychiatric nursing, the practitioner translates theory into living dialogue, guiding patients toward self-awareness and transformation. To practice psychotherapy is to engage in an evolving relationship that reflects trust, empathy, and shared humanity.

Among the most enduring conceptual frameworks influencing contemporary psychotherapy are developmental and attachment theories. These models explain how early relational experiences shape personality organization and emotional regulation. From infancy, the caregiver's responsiveness establishes internal working models of security or insecurity. When attachment needs are met consistently, the child develops trust, self-worth, and the capacity to form healthy bonds. When care is inconsistent, neglectful, or abusive, internal schemas of danger and shame emerge, predisposing to anxiety, depression, and interpersonal instability.

The PMHNP applies attachment theory to understand adult behavior and to create a reparative therapeutic environment. By modeling reliability, empathy, and emotional containment, the practitioner becomes a secure base from which the patient can explore vulnerable experiences. Over time, the patient learns that closeness does not inevitably lead to rejection or harm. This corrective experience rewires emotional learning at both psychological and neurobiological levels, validating that psychotherapy literally reshapes the brain through safe connection.

Developmental theory further extends across the lifespan. Erikson's psychosocial stages offer a valuable lens for clinical formulation, highlighting unresolved conflicts between autonomy and shame, industry and inferiority, or intimacy and isolation. A patient presenting with chronic self-doubt may still be struggling with mastery versus failure from earlier life phases. The PMHNP uses developmental assessment to tailor interventions to the individual's emotional age rather than chronological age, thereby enhancing engagement and outcome.

Trauma recovery within psychotherapy represents a particularly vital domain of practice. The PMHNP must recognize how trauma fragments memory, distorts identity, and embeds hyperarousal within the body. The therapeutic process unfolds in phases: establishing safety, processing traumatic memory, and integrating recovery into daily life. Safety involves stabilizing symptoms through grounding and mindfulness before delving into trauma narratives. Without this foundation, revisiting trauma risks reactivation and retraumatization. When safety and trust are established, trauma processing can occur through evidence-supported modalities such as Eye Movement Desensitization and Reprocessing, cognitive processing therapy, or somatic integration approaches. The nurse practitioner's calm presence, attuned listening, and careful pacing are as therapeutic as any technique. Healing trauma requires patience and respect for the survivor's autonomy; progress often emerges in nonlinear patterns marked by both breakthroughs and regressions.

Psychotherapy and pharmacotherapy frequently coexist in advanced practice. The PMHNP balances biological and psychological interventions so that each reinforces the other. Medication alleviates acute symptoms and creates cognitive space for insight, while therapy deepens understanding and addresses meaning. For example, antidepressants may lift mood sufficiently for a patient to engage in cognitive restructuring or relationship repair. The nurse practitioner ensures coherence between modalities, explaining that medication alters brain chemistry while therapy transforms neural pathways through new learning. Both processes are biological in nature; both depend on trust and commitment.

The therapeutic use of self remains the central instrument in all psychotherapeutic work. Self-awareness allows the practitioner to engage authentically without overidentification. Empathy must be disciplined, not indulgent. The PMHNP learns to sense the emotional atmosphere of the session, respond intuitively, and simultaneously observe the process analytically. The ability to tolerate silence, ambiguity, and emotional intensity distinguishes advanced practitioners from novices. Through presence alone—steady voice, calm posture, unwavering respect—the PMHNP conveys containment, offering patients an experience of stability often missing from their lives.

Supervision and continuous reflection are vital to sustaining therapeutic competence. Regular consultation with peers or supervisors provides a mirror to the clinician's internal world, revealing blind spots and countertransference dynamics that can cloud judgment. Reflective practice transforms emotional fatigue into insight, renewing the capacity for compassion. The disciplined therapist continually examines motivation, ethical responsibility, and the impact of personal values on clinical decisions.

Ethical and cultural sensitivity permeate every psychotherapeutic encounter. In a multicultural society, the PMHNP must recognize how race, gender, faith, socioeconomic status, and language shape identity and healing. The therapeutic space should be inclusive and respectful of difference. Cultural humility replaces assumptions of expertise with curiosity and openness. When the practitioner acknowledges limitations and invites collaboration, the alliance strengthens. The ethical mandate extends to advocacy for equitable access to care and to dismantling stigma associated with mental illness. The clinician embodies social responsibility, affirming the dignity and worth of every person served.

As therapy progresses, the termination phase becomes an integral component of healing. Ending therapy is not a simple conclusion but a developmental milestone representing autonomy and mastery. The PMHNP reviews accomplishments, reinforces internalized skills, and anticipates future challenges. Some patients experience sadness or anxiety at closure; the practitioner validates these feelings and interprets them as natural expressions of attachment and growth. By modeling healthy separation, the clinician helps the patient internalize a sense of enduring connection and self-reliance.

Psychotherapy also serves as a preventive and developmental tool, not merely a corrective one. Increasingly, individuals seek therapy to enhance self-knowledge, creativity, and emotional intelligence. The PMHNP recognizes that mental health is more than the absence of illness; it is the presence of integration, adaptability, and purpose. Therapy fosters these qualities by facilitating honest self-reflection and authentic living.

Ultimately, psychotherapy within advanced nursing practice exemplifies the profession's holistic philosophy. It bridges scientific understanding with compassionate presence, acknowledging the interplay of mind, body, and spirit. Each session becomes a microcosm of the healing process: assessment of suffering, creation of meaning, and cultivation of hope. The PMHNP emerges as a guide and witness, accompanying patients through the complex terrain of human emotion toward restoration and resilience.

Psychotherapy thus completes the circle of modern psychiatric care. It integrates the empirical precision of science with the transformative power of relationship. In the therapeutic space, both practitioner and patient engage in the timeless act of rehumanization—the rediscovery of coherence, dignity, and the capacity to love and to be loved. This is not only the essence of effective psychotherapy but also the embodiment of the nursing ideal itself.

Chapter 5: Ethics, Legal Principles, and Cultural Care

Ethical and legal competence form the cornerstone of psychiatric–mental health nurse practitioner practice. Every clinical decision reflects not only technical skill but moral reasoning. Ethics in mental health care transcends compliance; it represents a continual negotiation between compassion, justice, and respect for autonomy. The PMHNP must integrate professional codes, legal mandates, and cultural understanding to provide care that is safe, equitable, and dignified.

Ethical reasoning begins with awareness of the core principles that guide health care: beneficence, nonmaleficence, autonomy, justice, and fidelity. Beneficence calls the practitioner to act in the best interest of the patient; nonmaleficence warns against harm. Autonomy affirms the individual's right to make decisions about personal care, while justice demands fairness and equality in treatment. Fidelity encompasses honesty, faithfulness, and confidentiality within the therapeutic relationship. These principles rarely operate in isolation; they often conflict, requiring the PMHNP to engage in reflective judgment and to prioritize compassion guided by evidence and law.

One of the most pervasive ethical challenges in psychiatric nursing arises in the tension between autonomy and safety. A patient experiencing severe psychosis or suicidal intent may lack capacity to make informed choices. In such cases, the PMHNP must balance respect for freedom with the obligation to protect life. Involuntary treatment, though sometimes necessary, must always remain the last resort. The practitioner documents the reasoning process carefully, ensures procedural safeguards, and treats the patient with dignity throughout. Ethical intervention is measured not only by legal justification but by the preservation of trust and empathy even amid coercion.

Informed consent anchors all ethical practice. The PMHNP has the duty to ensure that consent is voluntary, informed, and competent. This process extends beyond a signature on a form; it is an ongoing dialogue that includes explanation of diagnosis, treatment options, potential benefits and risks, and alternatives. The nurse practitioner gauges comprehension by inviting the patient to restate information in personal words. In cases of diminished capacity, consent is obtained from legally authorized representatives, yet the patient's preferences and values remain central. Informed consent also applies to psychotherapy, pharmacologic treatment, and the sharing of clinical information. Transparency cultivates trust, reinforcing the ethical bond between clinician and patient.

Confidentiality represents another vital ethical and legal pillar. Psychiatric patients, whose disclosures often involve intimate or stigmatizing material, must trust that their information is protected. The Health Insurance Portability and Accountability Act (HIPAA) and corresponding state statutes delineate standards for data privacy. The PMHNP ensures secure record keeping, cautious communication, and discretion in public spaces. Exceptions to confidentiality—such as duty to warn or report abuse—require judicious interpretation. When disclosure becomes necessary to prevent serious harm, the practitioner limits the information shared to what is strictly relevant, informing the patient whenever possible. Ethical transparency transforms potential breaches into acts of responsibility rather than betrayal.

Boundaries define the integrity of professional relationships. The PMHNP occupies a position of power that demands vigilance against misuse. Overinvolvement, self-disclosure, or dual relationships risk distorting the therapeutic alliance. Boundaries protect both clinician and patient by maintaining clarity of purpose and professional distance. Yet therapeutic warmth and authenticity remain essential; the art lies in balancing accessibility with structure. Boundary maintenance extends into the digital realm—social media contact, texting, or informal communication blur professional lines. The conscientious practitioner establishes clear expectations regarding communication channels and availability, reinforcing ethical consistency.

Cultural competence transforms ethics into lived practice. To care for individuals from diverse backgrounds requires humility, self-examination, and continuous learning. Cultural competence is not static knowledge of customs but an attitude of openness to difference. The PMHNP recognizes how culture shapes perception of illness, help-seeking behavior, and expression of distress. A symptom interpreted as delusion in one context may represent a spiritual experience in another. Cultural humility means asking before assuming, listening before interpreting. The therapeutic encounter becomes a partnership of mutual discovery where both practitioner and patient learn.

Language access represents an ethical imperative. When linguistic barriers exist, the PMHNP ensures qualified interpreters rather than relying on family members, preserving confidentiality and accuracy. Cultural assessment includes exploration of family roles, communication style, and spiritual belief systems. In cross-cultural therapy, the clinician's willingness to acknowledge uncertainty fosters trust more effectively than feigned expertise.

Legal literacy empowers ethical practice. The PMHNP must remain informed about federal and state regulations governing scope of practice, prescriptive authority, record documentation, and involuntary commitment. Understanding malpractice elements—duty, breach, causation, and harm—reduces legal vulnerability. Documentation serves as the primary defense in legal scrutiny; clear, factual notes reflecting assessment, reasoning, and patient education demonstrate accountability.

The duty to protect and report constitutes a recurrent ethical tension. When a patient threatens identifiable others, the clinician may have a legal obligation to warn potential victims or law enforcement. Similarly, suspicion of child, elder, or dependent adult abuse mandates reporting to appropriate agencies. Such duties supersede confidentiality but must be executed with discretion and empathy. The PMHNP explains the rationale to the patient whenever feasible, emphasizing safety and ethical duty rather than punitive intent.

Justice and advocacy are inseparable from psychiatric ethics. Mental illness carries social stigma that limits access to housing, employment, and healthcare. The PMHNP acts as advocate not only for individuals but for communities marginalized by systemic inequities. Advocacy may involve policy participation, education, or public awareness initiatives that humanize mental health issues. At the clinical level, justice means allocating time, attention, and respect equitably across patients regardless of socioeconomic or cultural background.

Cultural care further extends into understanding collective trauma, migration, and historical oppression. The PMHNP acknowledges that mental health exists within sociopolitical context. Cultural safety arises when patients feel seen and valued within their own cultural narrative, free from microaggression or stereotyping. The practitioner cultivates an environment where diverse identities are affirmed. This includes sensitivity to gender, sexuality, and intersectional identities that influence mental well-being.

Ethical decision-making in advanced practice benefits from structured reflection. When faced with moral conflict, the PMHNP identifies stakeholders, clarifies values, explores options, and seeks consultation. Ethical committees, legal counsel, and peer supervision provide perspective that guards against impulsive or unilateral decisions. Documenting the deliberative process evidences professionalism and accountability.

Within interdisciplinary teams, ethical communication ensures cohesive care. The PMHNP shares necessary information for collaboration while safeguarding patient confidentiality. Respectful dialogue across disciplines models integrity and prevents fragmentation. Ethical leadership within teams fosters cultures of safety where staff feel empowered to voice concerns and reflect on moral challenges.

In the realm of research and evidence-based practice, ethics demands rigorous protection of participants and transparency in data reporting. The PMHNP engaging in research or quality improvement initiatives ensures informed consent, confidentiality, and honest interpretation of findings. Academic integrity reinforces public trust in nursing science.

Finally, self-care emerges as an ethical responsibility. The PMHNP who neglects personal well-being risks impaired judgment and compassion fatigue. Ethical codes recognize the clinician's obligation to maintain health sufficient for safe practice. Reflection, boundaries, supervision, and restorative activities sustain professional longevity and empathy. The ethical practitioner honors self and patient alike as equal participants in healing.

Ethics and law intertwine to form the moral architecture of psychiatric nursing. Through adherence to these principles, the PMHNP preserves the sacred trust of those who seek care. Ethical practice does not exist in abstraction; it is enacted in the ordinary gestures of respect, confidentiality, and informed partnership. The advanced psychiatric nurse practitioner, grounded in both law and compassion, transforms ethical ideals into daily acts of justice and care.

Forensic Ethics in Psychiatric Nursing

Forensic psychiatry intersects with ethics when mental health professionals work within legal contexts. The PMHNP may be called upon to provide evaluations of competence, criminal responsibility, or risk assessment in both civil and criminal legal proceedings. Ethical and legal awareness is paramount in these situations, as psychiatric evaluations can significantly influence a person's legal outcome.

In criminal law, the PMHNP might assess a defendant's mental state at the time of an offense, determining whether they were capable of understanding the nature of their actions or conforming to the law. This assessment must be objective, thorough, and unbiased, grounded in scientific principles and informed by established diagnostic criteria. The concept of mens rea, or the "guilty mind," shapes the clinician's understanding of criminal responsibility.

The ethical issue in forensic evaluations is the dual role of the clinician. The PMHNP must balance professional responsibilities to the patient with the legal obligation to provide an impartial assessment. This requires transparency about the evaluation's purpose and the limits of confidentiality. The practitioner must explain that the information shared will be used in a legal context, often without the same protections as a therapeutic conversation.

In cases involving involuntary commitment or civil competency, the PMHNP must act in accordance with state laws regarding the criteria for mental illness, risk of harm, and capacity to make decisions. The due process protections for individuals in the legal system demand that the PMHNP ensures all evaluations are conducted fairly and with respect for the individual's rights, even when the outcome may involve restriction of personal freedoms.

Ethical challenges also arise when working with incarcerated populations. Prisoners are at higher risk for mental health disorders, yet they often face barriers to care such as limited resources, stigma, and fear of retribution. The PMHNP must advocate for access to necessary treatments and ensure that their actions align with both medical ethics and correctional facility policies. Care for this population requires sensitivity to issues of coercion and the potential for psychological harm, which can distort patient–clinician relationships.

Cultural Care and Its Impact on Mental Health

Cultural care is an essential aspect of ethical psychiatric practice, especially as the PMHNP engages with increasingly diverse patient populations. Culture shapes every aspect of the patient's world: their worldview, coping mechanisms, expression of distress, and trust in healthcare systems. To be effective, the PMHNP must develop cultural humility—the recognition that no matter how much knowledge one gains, culture is always evolving, and no clinician can fully know all aspects of another person's cultural experience.

In clinical practice, the PMHNP asks, "What does mental health look like for this patient in the context of their culture?" This question allows the practitioner to understand symptoms through the lens of cultural meaning rather than pathologizing behaviors that are simply culturally unfamiliar. For example, neurasthenia in Chinese culture or susto in Latinx communities may reflect cultural expressions of distress that may be misunderstood if interpreted solely through the Western psychiatric framework. These culturally specific expressions of mental illness may not always align with DSM-5 criteria but still require compassionate and informed care.

Additionally, traditional healing practices and belief systems must be respected. The PMHNP integrates cultural care by inquiring about alternative therapies, spiritual beliefs, and family involvement. Collaboration with traditional healers or spiritual leaders may be an essential part of a comprehensive treatment plan. The practitioner's role is to create a space where patients can reconcile conventional and traditional treatments without judgment, all while ensuring that safety is maintained through informed consent and evidence-based guidelines.

The PMHNP must also be aware of intersectionality, recognizing that cultural identities are not monolithic. Gender, socioeconomic status, sexual orientation, and immigration status all influence a person's mental health and how they experience healthcare. For instance, an immigrant may face trauma related to their journey, compounded by acculturation stress. An individual who identifies as LGBTQIA+ may experience unique mental health challenges such as discrimination, family rejection, or internalized stigma. In these instances, culturally competent care involves recognizing these intersecting factors and responding in ways that affirm the patient's experience while providing effective treatment.

Global Health Ethics and Mental Health Care

In the broader context of global health, the ethical considerations of psychiatric care expand to encompass human rights, equity, and access to mental health services. The World Health Organization (WHO) recognizes mental health as a fundamental human right, yet in many parts of the world, mental health care is underfunded and neglected. The PMHNP's role as an advocate is critical in addressing disparities in global mental health.

Globally, mental health systems vary widely in terms of availability, cultural attitudes, and stigma. In low-resource settings, mental health care is often restricted to urban centers, leaving rural areas underserved. The PMHNP must understand and navigate these inequities, advocating for policy changes that promote access to care. Furthermore, the PMHNP might collaborate with international health organizations, governmental bodies, or non-governmental organizations (NGOs) to provide mental health services in underserved communities, ensuring that these services are culturally appropriate and accessible.

Ethical challenges in global health often arise when Western models of psychiatric care are imposed in settings where they are not culturally appropriate or feasible. The PMHNP must balance the desire to provide care with cultural humility, considering how local populations conceptualize mental illness and what treatments are acceptable to them.

Humanitarian crises, such as refugee situations, natural disasters, and armed conflicts, often result in significant mental health burdens. The PMHNP may be called to provide care to individuals who have experienced trauma, displacement, and loss. This care requires understanding of the unique ethical dilemmas posed by working with vulnerable populations, such as ensuring confidentiality in volatile settings, protecting vulnerable individuals from exploitation, and addressing the psychological needs of those who may not have access to adequate healthcare.

Leadership in Culturally Competent Systems of Care

Leadership in culturally competent care goes beyond direct patient care; it extends to creating systems that support and sustain diversity and inclusion. As leaders, the PMHNP must model cultural competence, advocate for patients, and challenge systems that perpetuate disparities in care. Organizational leadership involves the establishment of policies that ensure all staff are trained in cultural competence, recognize biases, and provide equitable care regardless of a patient's background.

At the clinical level, the PMHNP ensures that patients from diverse backgrounds feel welcomed, valued, and understood. This involves implementing systems of care that are linguistically accessible, culturally appropriate, and sensitive to the varied experiences of patients. From the initial intake process to treatment planning, leadership requires a continuous commitment to these principles. The PMHNP might lead initiatives to hire bilingual staff, offer culturally specific patient education materials, and develop support networks for minority populations.

Effective leadership in culturally competent care also includes a commitment to reducing health disparities within communities. By identifying gaps in services, advocating for policy changes, and participating in community education, the PMHNP helps create a culture of mental health that is inclusive and equitable. This work is vital in closing the treatment gap for underserved groups, ensuring that no patient is left behind because of their cultural or socioeconomic status.

Ethical Issues in Culturally Diverse Populations

Culturally diverse populations present unique ethical challenges that require careful consideration. One ethical issue is cultural relativism, which posits that moral values and practices should be understood in their cultural context. While it is essential to respect cultural differences, the PMHNP must navigate the line between cultural respect and ensuring patient safety. For example, traditional practices such as healing rituals, dietary restrictions, or family interventions may conflict with evidence-based medical practices. In these cases, the PMHNP must engage in respectful dialogue, advocating for safe and effective treatments while respecting the patient's cultural beliefs.

Another ethical issue arises in family-centered care, particularly in cultures where family plays a central role in decision-making. While family involvement is beneficial, it may conflict with the patient's autonomy, especially if the family is making decisions on behalf of a patient who desires more personal control over their care. In these situations, the PMHNP must balance respect for family dynamics with the individual's right to self-determination. This requires clear communication and careful navigation of the therapeutic relationship.

Finally, resource allocation becomes an ethical issue in many multicultural settings, especially where access to care is limited. The PMHNP may be faced with decisions regarding which patients receive priority for treatment or resources, based on urgency, vulnerability, or availability of services. These decisions require transparency, fairness, and a commitment to justice in mental health care.

Chapter 6: Practice Questions

Question (1-100)

Q1. A patient with major depressive disorder reports persistent low mood, loss of interest in activities, fatigue, and difficulty concentrating for the past two months. Which neurotransmitter imbalance is most strongly associated with these depressive symptoms?

(A) Reduced serotonin and norepinephrine
(B) Increased acetylcholine activity
(C) Increased glutamate inhibition
(D) Increased mesolimbic dopamine activity

Q2. A psychiatric nurse practitioner evaluates a patient who reports excessive worry about multiple life circumstances for more than six months along with muscle tension and sleep disturbance. Which diagnosis best fits this presentation?

(A) Social anxiety disorder
(B) Panic disorder
(C) Obsessive-compulsive disorder
(D) Generalized anxiety disorder

Q3. A patient taking lithium for bipolar disorder presents with tremor, nausea, diarrhea, and confusion. Which action is the most appropriate initial intervention?

(A) Stop lithium and obtain a serum lithium level
(B) Encourage increased caffeine intake
(C) Administer another dose of lithium
(D) Provide a benzodiazepine immediately

Q4. A patient with schizophrenia reports hearing voices that comment on his behavior even when no one is present. What type of symptom does this represent?

(A) Positive symptom
(B) Cognitive symptom
(C) Affective symptom
(D) Negative symptom

Q5. During a psychiatric interview, a patient suddenly stops speaking in the middle of a sentence and appears unable to recall what they were saying. Which thought process disturbance is being demonstrated?

(A) Circumstantiality
(B) Thought blocking
(C) Perseveration
(D) Flight of ideas

Q6. A patient diagnosed with bipolar I disorder is currently experiencing decreased need for sleep, grandiosity, and excessive goal-directed activity for one week. Which mood episode is most consistent with these findings?

(A) Major depressive episode
(B) Hypomanic episode
(C) Manic episode
(D) Cyclothymic episode

Q7. A patient with panic disorder experiences sudden episodes of intense fear accompanied by palpitations, sweating, and shortness of breath. What is the typical duration of a panic attack?

(A) Entire day
(B) 5-20 minutes
(C) Several hours

(D) A few seconds

Q8. A patient taking clozapine reports fever, sore throat, and fatigue. Which laboratory test should be obtained immediately?

(A) Thyroid stimulating hormone level
(B) Serum potassium level
(C) Complete blood count with differential
(D) Liver function tests

Q9. A patient repeatedly checks door locks dozens of times before leaving home despite knowing the behavior is excessive. Which disorder is most likely present?

(A) Somatic symptom disorder
(B) Panic disorder
(C) Post-traumatic stress disorder
(D) Obsessive-compulsive disorder

Q10. A patient with alcohol use disorder abruptly stops drinking and develops tremors, agitation, and sweating within 8 hours. Which medication is first-line for managing these withdrawal symptoms?

(A) Diazepam
(B) Lithium
(C) Fluoxetine
(D) Haloperidol

Q11. A patient persistently believes coworkers are plotting to harm him despite lack of evidence. Which type of delusion is most consistent with this belief?

(A) Nihilistic delusion
(B) Grandiose delusion
(C) Somatic delusion
(D) Persecutory delusion

Q12. A patient with borderline personality disorder demonstrates unstable relationships, impulsivity, and intense fear of abandonment. Which therapeutic approach has the strongest evidence for treatment?

(A) Psychoanalysis
(B) Dialectical behavior therapy
(C) Electroconvulsive therapy
(D) Hypnosis

Q13. A patient presents with persistent intrusive memories, nightmares, and hypervigilance three months after surviving a severe car accident. Which disorder best explains these symptoms?

(A) Acute stress disorder
(B) Generalized anxiety disorder
(C) Adjustment disorder
(D) Post-traumatic stress disorder

Q14. A patient demonstrates pressured speech, racing thoughts, and distractibility during the mental status examination. These findings most strongly suggest dysfunction in which neurotransmitter system?

(A) Histamine
(B) Dopamine
(C) GABA
(D) Acetylcholine

Q15. A patient taking selective serotonin reuptake inhibitors develops agitation, confusion, hyperreflexia, and diaphoresis. Which condition should be suspected?

(A) Lithium toxicity

(B) Serotonin syndrome
(C) Neuroleptic malignant syndrome
(D) Anticholinergic toxicity

Q16. A patient persistently collects items of little value and refuses to discard them, resulting in clutter that interferes with living spaces. Which diagnosis is most appropriate?
(A) Somatic symptom disorder
(B) Conversion disorder
(C) Cyclothymic disorder
(D) Hoarding disorder

Q17. A patient with schizophrenia shows diminished emotional expression, limited speech, and lack of motivation. These features represent which category of symptoms?
(A) Negative symptoms
(B) Dissociative symptoms
(C) Cognitive symptoms
(D) Positive symptoms

Q18. A patient presents with sudden blindness after a stressful event, but neurological examination and imaging reveal no physical cause. Which condition is most likely?
(A) Somatic symptom disorder
(B) Conversion disorder
(C) Illness anxiety disorder
(D) Factitious disorder

Q19. A patient complains of persistent fatigue, increased appetite, and excessive sleep during depressive episodes that occur mainly during winter months. Which diagnosis best fits this pattern?
(A) Premenstrual dysphoric disorder
(B) Major depressive disorder with seasonal pattern
(C) Persistent depressive disorder
(D) Cyclothymic disorder

Q20. A patient abruptly stops taking long-term benzodiazepine therapy and develops anxiety, tremors, and insomnia. What is the primary cause of these symptoms?
(A) Serotonin excess
(B) Central nervous system hyperexcitability
(C) Increased acetylcholine activity
(D) Dopamine depletion

Q21. A patient with schizophrenia begins taking haloperidol and develops severe muscle rigidity, fever, and altered mental status. Which condition should be suspected?
(A) Neuroleptic malignant syndrome
(B) Anticholinergic toxicity
(C) Lithium toxicity
(D) Serotonin syndrome

Q22. A patient reports experiencing intense fear when speaking in front of groups and avoids social situations due to fear of embarrassment. Which disorder is most consistent with these symptoms?
(A) Specific phobia
(B) Social anxiety disorder
(C) Panic disorder
(D) Generalized anxiety disorder

Q23. A patient taking monoamine oxidase inhibitors consumes aged cheese and later develops severe headache and elevated blood pressure. What complication has most likely occurred?
(A) Hypertensive crisis

(B) Serotonin toxicity
(C) Neuroleptic malignant syndrome
(D) Acute renal failure

Q24. A patient repeatedly interrupts others during conversations and shifts rapidly from one topic to another without completing thoughts. Which speech pattern is being demonstrated?
(A) Tangentiality
(B) Echolalia
(C) Circumstantiality
(D) Flight of ideas

Q25. A patient reports persistent feelings of emptiness, unstable relationships, and recurrent self-harm behaviors. Which personality disorder is most likely present?
(A) Borderline personality disorder
(B) Antisocial personality disorder
(C) Avoidant personality disorder
(D) Narcissistic personality disorder

Q26. A patient experiencing a manic episode sleeps only two hours per night but reports feeling energetic and rested. Which symptom is being demonstrated?
(A) Decreased need for sleep
(B) Circadian rhythm disorder
(C) Hypersomnia
(D) Insomnia disorder

Q27. A patient persistently believes their internal organs are rotting despite medical reassurance and normal tests. Which type of delusion does this represent?
(A) Grandiose delusion
(B) Somatic delusion
(C) Erotomanic delusion
(D) Referential delusion

Q28. A patient describes feeling detached from their own body as though observing themselves from outside. Which dissociative symptom is being described?
(A) Derealization
(B) Fugue state
(C) Depersonalization
(D) Dissociative amnesia

Q29. A patient displays excessive admiration for themselves and expects special treatment from others. Which personality disorder best fits this pattern?
(A) Schizoid personality disorder
(B) Dependent personality disorder
(C) Narcissistic personality disorder
(D) Paranoid personality disorder

Q30. A patient reports hearing a voice commenting on their actions while alone in a room. What type of hallucination is being described?
(A) Olfactory hallucination
(B) Auditory hallucination
(C) Visual hallucination
(D) Tactile hallucination

Q31. A patient repeatedly washes their hands dozens of times each day to relieve anxiety about contamination. Which term best describes this behavior?
(A) Obsession

(B) Compulsion
(C) Delusion
(D) Hallucination

Q32. A patient taking antipsychotic medication develops involuntary facial grimacing and tongue movements after several months of treatment. Which condition is most likely?

(A) Dystonia
(B) Parkinsonism
(C) Akathisia
(D) Tardive dyskinesia

Q33. A patient becomes extremely restless after starting a new antipsychotic medication and reports an inability to sit still. Which extrapyramidal symptom is most likely present?

(A) Tardive dyskinesia
(B) Dystonia
(C) Akathisia
(D) Parkinsonism

Q34. A patient reports believing that television messages are directed specifically at them. Which delusion type is being demonstrated?

(A) Persecutory delusion
(B) Delusion of reference
(C) Grandiose delusion
(D) Nihilistic delusion

Q35. A patient experiences persistent sadness for more than two years without periods of full recovery. Which diagnosis is most appropriate?

(A) Persistent depressive disorder
(B) Adjustment disorder
(C) Cyclothymic disorder
(D) Major depressive disorder

Q36. A patient with schizophrenia shows minimal facial expression and limited emotional response during conversation. Which term describes this presentation?

(A) Euphoric mood
(B) Expansive affect
(C) Labile affect
(D) Blunted affect

Q37. A patient begins experiencing tremors, rigidity, and slowed movement after starting an antipsychotic medication. Which extrapyramidal symptom is present?

(A) Dystonia
(B) Akathisia
(C) Parkinsonism
(D) Tardive dyskinesia

Q38. A patient suddenly develops painful muscle spasms of the neck and jaw after receiving an antipsychotic injection. Which condition is most likely?

(A) Serotonin syndrome
(B) Tardive dyskinesia
(C) Akathisia
(D) Acute dystonia

Q39. A patient demonstrates an exaggerated sense of self-importance and claims to possess extraordinary abilities. Which delusion is present?

(A) Referential delusion

(B) Somatic delusion
(C) Persecutory delusion
(D) Grandiose delusion

Q40. A patient with severe depression refuses to eat, speak, or move for prolonged periods. Which condition may best explain this presentation?
(A) Dissociation
(B) Somatization
(C) Delirium
(D) Catatonia

Q41. A patient hospitalized for severe depression reports hearing a voice telling them they are worthless and deserve punishment. Which specifier best describes this condition?
(A) Depression with psychotic features
(B) Adjustment disorder
(C) Depression with seasonal pattern
(D) Persistent depressive disorder

Q42. A patient frequently complains of physical symptoms such as headaches and stomach pain despite repeated normal medical evaluations. Which disorder is most consistent with this presentation?
(A) Conversion disorder
(B) Somatic symptom disorder
(C) Factitious disorder
(D) Illness anxiety disorder

Q43. A patient believes a famous celebrity is secretly in love with them despite no evidence. Which delusional subtype does this represent?
(A) Erotomanic delusion
(B) Nihilistic delusion
(C) Persecutory delusion
(D) Somatic delusion

Q44. A patient in therapy frequently shifts emotions rapidly from happiness to anger during a single session. Which affect pattern is being demonstrated?
(A) Blunted affect
(B) Restricted affect
(C) Flat affect
(D) Labile affect

Q45. A patient expresses persistent fear of leaving home because they believe escape would be difficult if panic symptoms occurred. Which condition is most likely present?
(A) Panic disorder without agoraphobia
(B) Social anxiety disorder
(C) Specific phobia
(D) Agoraphobia

Q46. A patient displays repetitive imitation of another person's movements during an examination. Which behavior is being demonstrated?
(A) Neologism
(B) Perseveration
(C) Echolalia
(D) Echopraxia

Q47. A patient repeatedly uses made-up words that have meaning only to them during conversation. Which speech disturbance is present?
(A) Neologism

(B) Echolalia
(C) Word salad
(D) Clang association

Q48. A patient describes feeling that the world around them seems unreal or dreamlike. Which dissociative experience does this represent?
(A) Dissociative amnesia
(B) Derealization
(C) Depersonalization
(D) Dissociative fugue

Q49. A patient becomes extremely fearful when encountering spiders and avoids places where spiders may be present. Which diagnosis is most appropriate?
(A) Generalized anxiety disorder
(B) Social anxiety disorder
(C) Panic disorder
(D) Specific phobia

Q50. A patient persistently forgets important personal information related to a traumatic event. Which dissociative disorder is most consistent with this symptom?
(A) Depersonalization disorder
(B) Conversion disorder
(C) Dissociative amnesia
(D) Dissociative identity disorder

Q51. A patient repeatedly returns to the same topic during conversation despite attempts to change the subject. Which thought process disturbance is present?
(A) Perseveration
(B) Tangentiality
(C) Flight of ideas
(D) Circumstantiality

Q52. A patient believes their thoughts are being removed from their mind by an external force. Which symptom is being described?
(A) Thought insertion
(B) Thought withdrawal
(C) Thought broadcasting
(D) Thought blocking

Q53. A patient insists that others can hear their thoughts without them speaking. Which symptom is present?
(A) Delusion of reference
(B) Thought insertion
(C) Thought broadcasting
(D) Thought blocking

Q54. A patient believes external forces are placing thoughts into their mind. Which symptom does this represent?
(A) Thought withdrawal
(B) Thought broadcasting
(C) Circumstantial thinking
(D) Thought insertion

Q55. A patient responds to questions with lengthy, unnecessary details but eventually returns to the main point. Which speech pattern is present?
(A) Circumstantiality

(B) Word salad
(C) Flight of ideas
(D) Tangentiality

Q56. A patient answers questions with responses that are unrelated and never return to the original topic. Which thought process is demonstrated?
(A) Tangentiality
(B) Circumstantiality
(C) Thought blocking
(D) Perseveration

Q57. A patient speaks using rhyming words with little logical meaning during conversation. Which speech pattern is present?
(A) Echolalia
(B) Neologism
(C) Clang association
(D) Circumstantiality

Q58. A patient with severe depression remains silent throughout the interview despite repeated questions. Which symptom is being demonstrated?
(A) Mutism
(B) Perseveration
(C) Echolalia
(D) Neologism

Q59. A patient displays exaggerated and dramatic emotional expression that appears theatrical during conversation. Which affect description best fits this presentation?
(A) Blunted affect
(B) Flat affect
(C) Expansive affect
(D) Restricted affect

Q60. A patient demonstrates incoherent speech consisting of unrelated words and phrases without meaningful structure. Which term best describes this speech pattern?
(A) Clang association
(B) Perseveration
(C) Word salad
(D) Neologism

Q61. A patient repeatedly echoes words spoken by the examiner during an interview. Which symptom is present?
(A) Clang association
(B) Echopraxia
(C) Echolalia
(D) Tangentiality

Q62. A patient insists that a major catastrophe will occur soon despite no supporting evidence. Which type of thinking pattern does this represent?
(A) Magical thinking
(B) Delusional thinking
(C) Catastrophic thinking
(D) Obsessive thinking

Q63. A patient believes that unrelated events are connected by hidden meanings meant specifically for them. Which symptom is present?
(A) Thought insertion

(B) Somatic delusion
(C) Grandiose delusion
(D) Delusion of reference

Q64. A patient experiences severe anxiety immediately after hearing a loud noise that reminds them of a previous traumatic event. Which phenomenon best explains this reaction?
(A) Conversion
(B) Conditioning
(C) Dissociation
(D) Hallucination

Q65. A patient suddenly begins wandering away from home and cannot recall their identity or past life events. Which disorder best explains this behavior?
(A) Dissociative amnesia
(B) Conversion disorder
(C) Depersonalization disorder
(D) Dissociative fugue

Q66. A patient with depression reports waking up several hours earlier than usual and being unable to return to sleep. Which sleep disturbance is present?
(A) Terminal insomnia
(B) Middle insomnia
(C) Hypersomnia
(D) Initial insomnia

Q67. A patient complains of persistent worry about having a serious illness despite repeated normal medical tests. Which diagnosis is most appropriate?
(A) Conversion disorder
(B) Somatic symptom disorder
(C) Factitious disorder
(D) Illness anxiety disorder

Q68. A patient with mania begins multiple ambitious projects but fails to complete them. Which symptom does this represent?
(A) Impulsivity
(B) Distractibility
(C) Psychomotor retardation
(D) Goal-directed activity

Q69. A patient believes their body has stopped functioning and that they are already dead. Which delusion type is present?
(A) Grandiose delusion
(B) Somatic delusion
(C) Nihilistic delusion
(D) Referential delusion

Q70. A patient demonstrates extremely rapid speech that is difficult to interrupt during an interview. Which speech pattern is present?
(A) Tangential speech
(B) Circumstantial speech
(C) Mutism
(D) Pressured speech

Q71. A patient describes sudden episodes of overwhelming fear accompanied by chest pain, dizziness, and a feeling of impending doom. Which condition is most consistent with this presentation?
(A) Adjustment disorder

(B) Social anxiety disorder
(C) Panic attack
(D) Generalized anxiety disorder

Q72. A patient reports difficulty initiating sleep despite feeling tired and spending hours in bed before falling asleep. Which sleep disturbance is present?

(A) Initial insomnia
(B) Terminal insomnia
(C) Hypersomnia
(D) Sleep paralysis

Q73. A patient appears drowsy during the interview but awakens easily when spoken to. Which level of consciousness best describes this state?

(A) Stuporous
(B) Lethargic
(C) Comatose
(D) Alert

Q74. A patient suddenly becomes unable to speak following a traumatic event despite no neurological damage. Which condition is most likely?

(A) Factitious disorder
(B) Illness anxiety disorder
(C) Dissociative identity disorder
(D) Conversion disorder

Q75. A patient persistently exaggerates physical symptoms to assume the role of a sick person without obvious external reward. Which disorder best fits this behavior?

(A) Somatic symptom disorder
(B) Malingering
(C) Factitious disorder
(D) Illness anxiety disorder

Q76. A patient intentionally exaggerates symptoms to obtain financial compensation. Which condition best describes this behavior?

(A) Malingering
(B) Conversion disorder
(C) Factitious disorder
(D) Somatic symptom disorder

Q77. A patient displays rigid adherence to rules, perfectionism, and excessive attention to detail that interferes with task completion. Which personality disorder is most likely?

(A) Antisocial personality disorder
(B) Narcissistic personality disorder
(C) Dependent personality disorder
(D) Obsessive-compulsive personality disorder

Q78. A patient refuses to make everyday decisions without excessive reassurance from others. Which personality disorder is most consistent with this behavior?

(A) Dependent personality disorder
(B) Avoidant personality disorder
(C) Paranoid personality disorder
(D) Schizoid personality disorder

Q79. A patient consistently avoids social interaction due to fear of criticism and feelings of inadequacy. Which personality disorder is most likely present?

(A) Borderline personality disorder

(B) Antisocial personality disorder
(C) Avoidant personality disorder
(D) Schizoid personality disorder

Q80. A patient shows little interest in forming close relationships and prefers solitary activities. Which personality disorder best fits this pattern?
(A) Schizoid personality disorder
(B) Paranoid personality disorder
(C) Histrionic personality disorder
(D) Dependent personality disorder

Q81. A patient consistently violates the rights of others, demonstrates deceitfulness, and lacks remorse for harmful behavior. Which personality disorder is most likely?
(A) Antisocial personality disorder
(B) Borderline personality disorder
(C) Paranoid personality disorder
(D) Narcissistic personality disorder

Q82. A patient believes others are constantly plotting against them and refuses to trust anyone. Which personality disorder best explains this pattern?
(A) Avoidant personality disorder
(B) Schizoid personality disorder
(C) Paranoid personality disorder
(D) Dependent personality disorder

Q83. A patient seeks constant attention and displays exaggerated emotional behavior during interactions. Which personality disorder is most consistent with this presentation?
(A) Histrionic personality disorder
(B) Narcissistic personality disorder
(C) Dependent personality disorder
(D) Borderline personality disorder

Q84. A patient expresses feelings of emptiness and frequently shifts between idealizing and devaluing others. Which personality disorder is most likely?
(A) Avoidant personality disorder
(B) Borderline personality disorder
(C) Schizoid personality disorder
(D) Dependent personality disorder

Q85. A patient demonstrates persistent elevated mood, increased energy, and inflated self-esteem lasting several days without severe impairment. Which episode best describes this presentation?
(A) Cyclothymic episode
(B) Hypomanic episode
(C) Manic episode
(D) Major depressive episode

Q86. A patient with bipolar disorder experiences alternating periods of hypomanic and mild depressive symptoms that persist for several years. Which diagnosis is most appropriate?
(A) Major depressive disorder
(B) Bipolar I disorder
(C) Cyclothymic disorder
(D) Persistent depressive disorder

Q87. A patient reports intense fear of gaining weight despite being underweight. Which eating disorder is most consistent with this presentation?
(A) Avoidant restrictive food intake disorder

(B) Anorexia nervosa
(C) Binge eating disorder
(D) Bulimia nervosa

Q88. A patient engages in recurrent binge eating followed by self-induced vomiting. Which eating disorder is most likely present?
(A) Pica
(B) Bulimia nervosa
(C) Anorexia nervosa
(D) Binge eating disorder

Q89. A patient consumes large amounts of food rapidly without compensatory behaviors and feels ashamed afterward. Which eating disorder best fits this description?
(A) Rumination disorder
(B) Binge eating disorder
(C) Bulimia nervosa
(D) Anorexia nervosa

Q90. A patient persistently eats non-nutritive substances such as clay or chalk. Which disorder best describes this behavior?
(A) Rumination disorder
(B) Binge eating disorder
(C) Pica
(D) Avoidant restrictive food intake disorder

Q91. A patient repeatedly regurgitates food shortly after eating and then re-chews or spits it out. Which disorder best explains this behavior?
(A) Rumination disorder
(B) Bulimia nervosa
(C) Pica
(D) Binge eating disorder

Q92. A patient persistently restricts food intake due to lack of interest in eating rather than fear of weight gain. Which disorder is most likely?
(A) Bulimia nervosa
(B) Binge eating disorder
(C) Avoidant restrictive food intake disorder
(D) Anorexia nervosa

Q93. A patient reports recurrent episodes of sleepwalking during which they leave bed and perform complex activities. Which disorder is most consistent with this description?
(A) Narcolepsy
(B) REM sleep behavior disorder
(C) Somnambulism
(D) Insomnia disorder

Q94. A patient suddenly experiences brief episodes of uncontrollable sleep during the day. Which disorder is most likely present?
(A) Insomnia disorder
(B) Narcolepsy
(C) Circadian rhythm disorder
(D) Sleep apnea

Q95. A patient reports loud snoring and frequent pauses in breathing during sleep. Which condition should be suspected?
(A) Narcolepsy

(B) Insomnia disorder
(C) Sleep terror disorder
(D) Obstructive sleep apnea

Q96. A child awakens suddenly during the night screaming and appearing terrified but cannot recall the episode in the morning. Which disorder is most consistent with this description?

(A) Narcolepsy
(B) Insomnia disorder
(C) Sleep terror disorder
(D) Nightmare disorder

Q97. A patient frequently experiences vivid frightening dreams that cause awakening and clear recall. Which condition best explains this symptom?

(A) Narcolepsy
(B) Nightmare disorder
(C) Somnambulism
(D) Sleep terror disorder

Q98. A patient experiences temporary inability to move while falling asleep or waking. Which condition is being described?

(A) Insomnia disorder
(B) Circadian rhythm disorder
(C) Sleep paralysis
(D) Narcolepsy

Q99. A patient works night shifts and struggles to sleep during the day while feeling excessively tired at work. Which disorder best explains this problem?

(A) Insomnia disorder
(B) Sleep apnea
(C) Narcolepsy
(D) Circadian rhythm sleep disorder

Q100. A patient experiences persistent difficulty falling asleep, staying asleep, or obtaining restorative sleep despite adequate opportunity. Which disorder is most consistent with this description?

(A) Insomnia disorder
(B) Sleep terror disorder
(C) Circadian rhythm disorder
(D) Narcolepsy

Answer Key and Explanation (1-100)

Q1. Answer: A

Explanation: Major depressive disorder is strongly associated with decreased levels of serotonin and norepinephrine in key brain pathways responsible for mood regulation. These neurotransmitters influence emotional stability, energy levels, motivation, and sleep patterns. When their levels are reduced, patients commonly experience sadness, fatigue, poor concentration, and anhedonia. Modern antidepressant therapies aim to increase the availability of these neurotransmitters in synaptic spaces. Restoring neurotransmitter balance can gradually improve mood and cognitive functioning. This neurochemical model explains why medications targeting serotonin and norepinephrine pathways are effective treatments for depression.

Q2. Answer: D

Explanation: Generalized anxiety disorder is characterized by persistent and excessive worry about a variety of everyday life situations. The worry occurs most days for at least six months and is difficult for the patient to control. Physical symptoms such as muscle tension, fatigue, irritability, restlessness, and sleep disturbances frequently accompany the condition. The anxiety is not limited to specific situations and often affects work, relationships, and daily functioning. Patients often describe feeling constantly on edge or unable to relax. Early recognition allows treatment through psychotherapy, lifestyle modification, and pharmacologic therapy when necessary.

Q3. Answer: A

Explanation: Lithium toxicity should be suspected when a patient taking lithium develops gastrointestinal symptoms, tremor, confusion, or neurological changes. The first priority is to discontinue the medication and evaluate the serum lithium concentration to determine severity. Lithium has a narrow therapeutic index, making toxicity a significant clinical concern. Early identification helps prevent progression to severe complications such as seizures or renal impairment. Monitoring renal function and hydration status is also essential during evaluation. Prompt management can reduce morbidity and prevent life-threatening outcomes.

Q4. Answer: A

Explanation: Positive symptoms refer to experiences that are added to normal mental functioning and are commonly seen in schizophrenia. These include hallucinations, delusions, disorganized speech, and abnormal behavior. Auditory hallucinations are the most common type and often involve voices commenting or conversing with the patient. Such symptoms reflect altered perception and distorted reality testing. They typically respond well to antipsychotic medications that modulate dopamine pathways. Early treatment can reduce symptom severity and improve overall functioning.

Q5. Answer: B

Explanation: Thought blocking occurs when a person suddenly stops speaking because their train of thought is abruptly interrupted. Patients often describe the experience as their mind going blank or losing the idea they were expressing. This phenomenon is commonly observed in psychotic disorders such as schizophrenia. It may also appear during severe anxiety or cognitive disturbance. The interruption can occur repeatedly during conversation and significantly impair communication. Careful observation of speech patterns during mental status examination helps identify this disturbance.

Q6. Answer: C

Explanation: A manic episode involves a distinct period of abnormally elevated, expansive, or irritable mood lasting at least one week. Symptoms often include decreased need for sleep, inflated self-esteem, grandiosity, increased goal-directed activity, and rapid speech. These symptoms are severe enough to cause marked impairment in functioning or require hospitalization. Mania is a defining feature of bipolar I disorder. Recognition of manic symptoms is important because untreated episodes can lead to risky behavior and psychosocial consequences. Treatment typically includes mood stabilizers and sometimes antipsychotic medications.

Q7. Answer: B

Explanation: Panic attacks are sudden episodes of intense fear that peak rapidly and typically last between five and twenty minutes. During this period, patients may experience physical symptoms such as heart palpitations, sweating, trembling, chest discomfort, and shortness of breath. Many individuals also feel a sense of impending doom or fear of losing control. Although the symptoms are intense, they usually resolve relatively quickly. Recurrent attacks can lead to avoidance behaviors and anticipatory anxiety. Early treatment often includes cognitive behavioral therapy and pharmacologic interventions when needed.

Q8. Answer: C

Explanation: Clozapine is associated with a risk of agranulocytosis, a potentially life-threatening reduction in neutrophils. Symptoms such as fever, sore throat, and fatigue may indicate developing infection due to compromised immune defense. Immediate evaluation with a complete blood count and differential is necessary to assess white blood cell and absolute neutrophil levels. Regular hematologic monitoring is required for all patients receiving this medication. Early detection allows prompt discontinuation and treatment to prevent severe complications. Monitoring programs have significantly improved the safety of clozapine therapy.

Q9. Answer: D

Explanation: Obsessive-compulsive disorder is characterized by intrusive thoughts or urges and repetitive behaviors performed to reduce anxiety. Patients often recognize that their behaviors are irrational but feel unable to resist performing them. Checking behaviors, such as repeatedly confirming that doors are locked, are common compulsions. These rituals temporarily relieve distress caused by obsessive fears. Over time the behavior can become time-consuming and interfere with daily functioning. Treatment commonly includes cognitive behavioral therapy and medications that increase serotonin activity.

Q10. Answer: A

Explanation: Benzodiazepines are the first-line treatment for alcohol withdrawal because they enhance inhibitory neurotransmission in the central nervous system. These medications help reduce symptoms such as tremors, agitation, anxiety, and risk of seizures. Alcohol withdrawal occurs due to neurochemical imbalance after sudden cessation of chronic alcohol intake. Without treatment, symptoms can progress to severe complications including delirium tremens. Benzodiazepines stabilize neurological activity and provide safe detoxification. Careful monitoring is required to adjust dosing and ensure patient safety.

Q11. Answer: D

Explanation: Persecutory delusions involve false beliefs that one is being harmed, harassed, or conspired against by others. Patients often interpret neutral events as threatening and may become suspicious of coworkers, neighbors, or family members. These beliefs remain fixed despite clear evidence to the contrary. Such delusions are common in psychotic disorders including schizophrenia and delusional disorder. They can significantly affect interpersonal relationships and daily functioning. Antipsychotic medications and supportive psychotherapy are often used to reduce symptom severity.

Q12. Answer: B

Explanation: Dialectical behavior therapy is a structured psychotherapy designed to treat individuals with severe emotional dysregulation and impulsive behaviors. It focuses on developing skills in mindfulness, emotional regulation, distress tolerance, and interpersonal effectiveness. The approach helps patients learn healthier coping strategies when experiencing intense emotions. It was originally developed specifically for individuals with borderline personality disorder. Research has demonstrated significant reductions in self-harm and suicidal behaviors with this treatment. Structured therapy programs often include both individual and group sessions.

Q13. Answer: D

Explanation: Post-traumatic stress disorder develops after exposure to a traumatic event and involves persistent re-experiencing of the trauma. Symptoms include intrusive memories, nightmares, emotional distress, avoidance behaviors, and heightened arousal. The condition is diagnosed when symptoms persist for more than one month following the traumatic event. Patients often experience hypervigilance, irritability, and sleep disturbance. Trauma reminders may trigger intense psychological distress. Effective treatments include trauma-focused psychotherapy and certain antidepressant medications.

Q14. Answer: B

Explanation: Dopamine dysregulation plays a central role in several psychiatric conditions including mania and psychosis. Increased dopaminergic activity can lead to heightened energy, rapid speech, and racing thoughts. These symptoms reflect overstimulation of neural circuits associated with reward and motivation. Excessive dopamine signaling may also contribute to impulsivity and impaired judgment. Many medications used to treat mania and psychosis work by reducing dopamine activity in specific brain pathways. Understanding neurotransmitter involvement helps guide pharmacologic treatment strategies.

Q15. Answer: B

Explanation: Serotonin syndrome occurs when excessive serotonin accumulates in the central nervous system. It often results from medication interactions or high doses of serotonergic drugs. Symptoms include agitation, confusion, hyperreflexia, muscle rigidity, and excessive sweating. The condition can develop rapidly and may become life-threatening if untreated. Immediate discontinuation of serotonergic medications is essential. Supportive care and specific medications may be required to control severe symptoms.

Q16. Answer: D

Explanation: Hoarding disorder involves persistent difficulty discarding possessions regardless of their actual value. Individuals often feel strong emotional attachment to items and experience distress when attempting to discard them. Over time, accumulation leads to cluttered living spaces that interfere with daily activities and safety. The behavior is not simply collecting but rather an inability to part with objects. The condition may cause social isolation and functional impairment. Treatment typically involves cognitive behavioral therapy aimed at improving decision-making and organization skills.

Q17. Answer: A

Explanation: Negative symptoms refer to deficits in normal emotional and behavioral functioning. These may include reduced emotional expression, diminished speech output, lack of motivation, and social withdrawal. Such symptoms can be more disabling than positive symptoms because they interfere with daily functioning and relationships. They are often resistant to treatment and may persist even when hallucinations or delusions improve. These features reflect reduced activity in neural circuits responsible for motivation and emotional responsiveness. Comprehensive treatment often requires psychosocial rehabilitation in addition to medication.

Q18. Answer: B

Explanation: Conversion disorder involves neurological symptoms that cannot be explained by medical evaluation. Symptoms may include paralysis, blindness, or seizures occurring after psychological stress. The symptoms are not intentionally produced and are believed to represent unconscious psychological conflict expressed physically. Patients often experience significant distress or impairment in functioning. Careful evaluation is necessary to rule out underlying medical conditions. Treatment typically includes psychotherapy focused on stress management and emotional processing.

Q19. Answer: B

Explanation: Major depressive disorder with seasonal pattern involves recurrent depressive episodes occurring during specific seasons, most commonly winter. Patients frequently report increased sleep, fatigue, carbohydrate cravings, and weight gain. Reduced exposure to natural sunlight may disrupt circadian rhythms and neurotransmitter regulation. These changes can influence mood and energy levels.

Symptoms usually improve when seasons change and daylight exposure increases. Treatments often include light therapy, psychotherapy, and antidepressant medications when necessary.

Q20. Answer: B

Explanation: Benzodiazepines enhance inhibitory neurotransmission in the central nervous system by acting on GABA receptors. When the medication is discontinued suddenly after prolonged use, the brain experiences a rebound increase in excitatory activity. This leads to symptoms such as anxiety, tremors, agitation, and sleep disturbance. In severe cases, seizures may occur due to excessive neuronal excitability. Gradual tapering of the medication is recommended to prevent withdrawal symptoms. Careful monitoring during dose reduction helps ensure patient safety and comfort.

Q21. Answer: A

Explanation: Neuroleptic malignant syndrome is a rare but life-threatening reaction associated with antipsychotic medications. It is characterized by severe muscle rigidity, hyperthermia, altered mental status, and autonomic instability. The condition results from abrupt dopamine blockade in the central nervous system. Early recognition is critical because untreated cases can lead to serious complications such as renal failure or cardiovascular collapse. Immediate discontinuation of the offending medication and supportive medical treatment are required. Intensive monitoring and prompt management significantly improve patient outcomes.

Q22. Answer: B

Explanation: Social anxiety disorder involves an intense fear of being negatively evaluated or embarrassed in social or performance situations. Individuals often avoid situations such as public speaking, meeting new people, or eating in public. The fear is disproportionate to the actual threat and can significantly interfere with daily functioning. Physical symptoms such as sweating, trembling, or rapid heart rate may occur during exposure to feared situations. The condition often develops during adolescence and may persist without treatment. Cognitive behavioral therapy and certain medications can effectively reduce symptoms.

Q23. Answer: A

Explanation: Monoamine oxidase inhibitors interfere with the breakdown of tyramine, a compound found in certain aged and fermented foods. When tyramine accumulates in the body, it can trigger a sudden and dangerous increase in blood pressure. This reaction is known as hypertensive crisis and can present with severe headache, sweating, palpitations, and elevated blood pressure. Without treatment, the condition may lead to stroke or other serious complications. Patients receiving these medications must follow strict dietary restrictions. Education about avoiding high-tyramine foods is essential for safe treatment.

Q24. Answer: D

Explanation: Flight of ideas involves rapid shifting from one topic to another with loosely connected associations. Although the ideas may still have some connection, the pace of thinking is accelerated and difficult to follow. This pattern is frequently observed during manic episodes in bipolar disorder. Patients often appear highly energetic and may speak rapidly with pressured speech. The fast flow of ideas reflects increased cognitive activity. Recognizing this pattern during assessment helps clinicians identify underlying mood disorders.

Q25. Answer: A

Explanation: Borderline personality disorder is characterized by emotional instability, impulsive behaviors, and unstable interpersonal relationships. Patients frequently report chronic feelings of emptiness and intense fear of abandonment. Self-harm behaviors such as cutting may occur during periods of emotional distress. Relationships often fluctuate between idealization and devaluation. Emotional responses may be intense and rapidly changing. Psychotherapeutic approaches focusing on emotional regulation and coping strategies are essential in treatment.

Q26. Answer: A

Explanation: Decreased need for sleep is a hallmark symptom of mania. Unlike insomnia, the patient does not feel fatigued despite sleeping very little. Individuals may remain active and energetic even after only a few hours of rest. This symptom often accompanies elevated mood, increased activity, and rapid thinking. It reflects heightened central nervous system stimulation. Recognizing this feature is important for identifying manic episodes in bipolar disorder.

Q27. Answer: B

Explanation: Somatic delusions involve false beliefs about bodily functions or physical health. Patients may believe their organs are damaged, infected, or deteriorating despite medical evidence to the contrary. These beliefs remain fixed and are not corrected by reassurance. Somatic delusions may occur in psychotic disorders or severe mood disorders. The belief often causes significant anxiety and distress. Antipsychotic medications and psychotherapy are commonly used to address these symptoms.

Q28. Answer: C

Explanation: Depersonalization involves a disturbing sense of detachment from one's own body or mental processes. Individuals may feel as though they are observing themselves from outside or functioning on autopilot. Despite the altered perception, reality testing remains intact. The experience is often associated with severe stress, trauma, or anxiety disorders. Episodes may be temporary or recurrent depending on the underlying cause. Treatment focuses on addressing the psychological stressors contributing to the condition.

Q29. Answer: C

Explanation: Narcissistic personality disorder involves a pervasive pattern of grandiosity and need for admiration. Individuals often exaggerate achievements and expect recognition without corresponding accomplishments. They may display a lack of empathy and exploit others to achieve personal goals. Relationships may suffer due to entitlement and arrogance. Despite outward confidence, underlying self-esteem may be fragile. Psychotherapy focuses on improving interpersonal awareness and emotional regulation.

Q30. Answer: B

Explanation: Auditory hallucinations involve hearing sounds or voices that are not present in the external environment. These experiences commonly occur in psychotic disorders such as schizophrenia. Voices may comment on the patient's actions, issue commands, or engage in conversation. The hallucinations often feel real and may influence behavior. Such symptoms reflect altered sensory perception and impaired reality testing. Antipsychotic medications are commonly used to reduce these experiences.

Q31. Answer: B

Explanation: Compulsions are repetitive behaviors performed in response to obsessive thoughts or anxiety. The behavior is intended to reduce distress or prevent a feared outcome. In obsessive-compulsive disorder, these actions often become excessive and time consuming. Hand washing is one of the most common compulsive behaviors related to contamination fears. Although the patient recognizes the behavior may be irrational, the urge to perform it is difficult to resist. Treatment usually includes cognitive behavioral therapy and medications affecting serotonin.

Q32. Answer: D

Explanation: Tardive dyskinesia is a movement disorder associated with long-term use of antipsychotic medications. It typically presents with repetitive, involuntary movements of the face, mouth, tongue, or limbs. These movements may include grimacing, lip smacking, or tongue protrusion. The condition results from chronic dopamine receptor blockade in the brain. Symptoms may persist even after the medication is discontinued. Early detection through routine monitoring can reduce the risk of permanent movement disorders.

Q33. Answer: C

Explanation: Akathisia is characterized by a subjective sense of inner restlessness and an inability to remain still. Patients may pace, shift weight frequently, or constantly move their legs. This condition often occurs shortly after starting or increasing the dose of antipsychotic medications. The discomfort can be severe and may increase risk of treatment noncompliance. Management often includes dose adjustment or medications that reduce the symptoms. Early identification is important for maintaining effective treatment.

Q34. Answer: B

Explanation: Delusions of reference involve the belief that neutral events or messages are directed specifically toward oneself. Individuals may interpret television broadcasts, songs, or newspaper articles as containing personal messages. This interpretation occurs despite lack of objective evidence. Such beliefs are commonly seen in psychotic disorders including schizophrenia. They reflect disturbances in perception and interpretation of environmental stimuli. Treatment focuses on addressing the underlying psychotic condition.

Q35. Answer: A

Explanation: Persistent depressive disorder involves a chronic depressed mood lasting at least two years in adults. Symptoms may be less severe than those seen in major depressive episodes but remain continuous over long periods. Individuals often experience low energy, poor self-esteem, and feelings of hopelessness. Because symptoms are long-standing, patients may view the mood as part of their personality. The condition can significantly impair functioning and quality of life. Treatment typically includes psychotherapy and antidepressant medications.

Q36. Answer: D

Explanation: Blunted affect refers to a noticeable reduction in emotional expression. Patients may speak in a monotone voice and display limited facial movements. Emotional responses appear diminished even when discussing significant events. This feature is commonly associated with negative symptoms of schizophrenia. It reflects decreased emotional responsiveness rather than absence of emotion. Recognition of affect changes is an important component of the mental status examination.

Q37. Answer: C

Explanation: Drug-induced parkinsonism resembles the symptoms seen in Parkinson's disease. Patients may develop tremors, muscle rigidity, and slowed movements after starting dopamine-blocking medications. These symptoms result from reduced dopamine activity in motor pathways. Antipsychotic medications commonly cause this effect, especially older agents. The condition can significantly affect mobility and daily functioning. Management may include medication adjustments or medications that restore dopamine balance.

Q38. Answer: D

Explanation: Acute dystonia is a sudden and often painful muscle contraction that occurs shortly after initiating antipsychotic medications. The spasms frequently affect muscles of the neck, jaw, tongue, or eyes. The condition can appear frightening to patients and may impair breathing or swallowing in severe cases. It results from sudden dopamine blockade affecting motor control pathways. Treatment usually involves medications that restore balance between neurotransmitter systems. Rapid intervention quickly relieves symptoms.

Q39. Answer: D

Explanation: Grandiose delusions involve false beliefs of exceptional abilities, wealth, or power. Patients may believe they possess unique talents or hold an important role in society. These beliefs remain fixed despite contradictory evidence. Grandiose thinking is frequently observed in manic episodes of bipolar disorder and certain psychotic conditions. The inflated self-perception may lead to risky decisions or unrealistic plans. Appropriate treatment focuses on stabilizing mood and addressing psychotic symptoms.

Q40. Answer: D

Explanation: Catatonia is a psychomotor syndrome characterized by abnormal movement or lack of movement. Patients may remain motionless, mute, or unresponsive for extended periods. It can occur in mood disorders, psychotic disorders, and certain medical conditions. In severe cases individuals may require medical support to maintain nutrition and hydration. Early recognition is important because effective treatments are available. Appropriate intervention often leads to rapid improvement in symptoms.

Q41. Answer: A

Explanation: Major depressive episodes can sometimes include psychotic symptoms when the illness becomes severe. Individuals may experience hallucinations or delusions that are often consistent with depressive themes such as guilt, punishment, or worthlessness. These symptoms reflect a significant disruption in perception and thinking. The presence of psychosis indicates a more severe form of depression and often requires more intensive treatment. Combined pharmacologic approaches using antidepressants and antipsychotics are frequently required. Early intervention helps prevent worsening of symptoms and improves recovery outcomes.

Q42. Answer: B

Explanation: Somatic symptom disorder involves persistent physical complaints that cause significant distress or impairment. The symptoms may or may not have a medical explanation, but the individual experiences excessive concern about them. Patients often seek repeated medical evaluations and reassurance. The focus on physical symptoms can dominate daily life and emotional functioning. Psychological stress frequently contributes to symptom intensity. Treatment focuses on building a supportive therapeutic relationship and addressing underlying emotional concerns.

Q43. Answer: A

Explanation: Erotomanic delusions involve the belief that another person, often someone famous or of higher status, is secretly in love with the individual. The belief persists despite clear evidence to the contrary. Patients may misinterpret ordinary events as confirmation of the imagined relationship. This condition is commonly associated with delusional disorder. The belief can sometimes lead to attempts to contact or pursue the perceived admirer. Treatment typically includes antipsychotic medication and supportive therapy.

Q44. Answer: D

Explanation: Labile affect refers to rapid and often exaggerated changes in emotional expression. Individuals may move quickly from laughter to tears or anger without clear triggers. These emotional shifts may occur within minutes or even seconds. Such patterns are commonly observed in certain mood disorders and personality disorders. The instability reflects difficulty regulating emotional responses. Identifying affect patterns during assessment helps guide diagnosis and treatment planning.

Q45. Answer: D

Explanation: Agoraphobia involves intense anxiety about situations where escape might be difficult or help unavailable if panic symptoms develop. Common fears include being in crowds, using public transportation, or leaving home alone. Individuals may avoid these situations or endure them with severe distress. Over time the avoidance behavior can significantly restrict daily activities. The condition frequently occurs alongside panic disorder but can also appear independently. Treatment typically includes cognitive behavioral therapy and sometimes medication.

Q46. Answer: D

Explanation: Echopraxia is the involuntary imitation of another person's movements or gestures. This behavior may occur in certain psychiatric and neurological conditions. It reflects impaired control of motor responses and abnormal social interaction patterns. The behavior may be subtle or obvious depending on the severity. Echopraxia is often associated with catatonia and certain psychotic disorders. Observing such behaviors during examination provides important diagnostic information.

Q47. Answer: A

Explanation: Neologisms are newly invented words or expressions that have meaning only to the individual using them. These words are often unintelligible to others and disrupt normal communication. Neologisms are commonly observed in severe thought disorders associated with psychotic illnesses. They reflect significant disturbances in language processing and cognitive organization. Identifying this speech pattern helps clinicians assess the severity of thought disorder. Appropriate treatment aims to reduce underlying psychotic symptoms.

Q48. Answer: B

Explanation: Derealization involves a sense that the external environment feels strange, unreal, or distorted. Individuals may describe the world as foggy, distant, or dreamlike. Despite the altered perception, the person remains aware that the experience is unusual. This symptom often occurs during episodes of severe anxiety or trauma. It represents a form of dissociation that temporarily separates perception from emotional experience. Treatment focuses on addressing the underlying psychological stress and improving coping skills.

Q49. Answer: D

Explanation: Specific phobia involves intense fear of a particular object or situation. The fear is disproportionate to the actual danger and leads to avoidance behavior. Common examples include fears of animals, heights, or flying. Exposure to the feared stimulus often triggers immediate anxiety or panic. The condition can interfere with daily functioning when avoidance behaviors become extensive. Behavioral therapies such as gradual exposure are highly effective treatments.

Q50. Answer: C

Explanation: Dissociative amnesia involves an inability to recall important personal information, usually related to stressful or traumatic events. The memory loss cannot be explained by ordinary forgetfulness or neurological conditions. Individuals may lose memories of specific events, time periods, or aspects of their identity. This psychological defense mechanism helps protect the person from overwhelming emotional distress. The condition may resolve spontaneously or with therapeutic intervention. Psychotherapy often helps individuals gradually recover and process lost memories.

Q51. Answer: A

Explanation: Perseveration refers to the persistent repetition of a particular thought, word, or topic. The individual continues returning to the same subject even when it is no longer relevant to the conversation. This pattern often reflects impaired cognitive flexibility. It can occur in various psychiatric and neurological conditions. The behavior may interfere with effective communication. Observing this pattern during interview helps clinicians identify cognitive or thought process disturbances.

Q52. Answer: B

Explanation: Thought withdrawal is the belief that one's thoughts are being taken away by an outside force. Patients may feel their mind suddenly becomes empty because someone has removed their thoughts. This phenomenon is considered a type of thought control delusion. It commonly occurs in psychotic disorders such as schizophrenia. The experience can cause significant distress and confusion. Antipsychotic medications are commonly used to treat these symptoms.

Q53. Answer: C

Explanation: Thought broadcasting involves the belief that one's thoughts are accessible to others. Patients may feel that people around them can hear or know what they are thinking. This belief represents a disturbance in the sense of mental privacy. It is commonly associated with psychotic disorders. The symptom reflects impaired boundaries between internal thoughts and the external world. Treatment focuses on addressing the underlying psychotic process.

Q54. Answer: D

Explanation: Thought insertion refers to the belief that thoughts are being placed into one's mind by an outside force. Patients may feel these thoughts do not belong to them. This experience reflects a loss of control over personal thinking processes. It is commonly observed in schizophrenia and other psychotic conditions. The symptom indicates severe disturbance in perception of self and cognition. Effective treatment often includes antipsychotic medication and supportive therapy.

Q55. Answer: A

Explanation: Circumstantiality involves providing excessive and unnecessary detail during conversation. The individual eventually reaches the original point but only after lengthy explanations. This pattern can make communication slow and difficult to follow. It differs from tangential thinking because the person ultimately returns to the main topic. Circumstantial speech may appear in certain mood disorders or cognitive disturbances. Careful observation helps clinicians differentiate among types of thought process abnormalities.

Q56. Answer: A

Explanation: Tangentiality occurs when responses to questions diverge from the topic and never return to the original point. The person's thinking becomes disconnected from the direction of the conversation. This pattern reflects impaired logical organization of thought. It is often observed in psychotic disorders and severe cognitive disturbances. Communication may become difficult because answers fail to address the question asked. Identifying this pattern helps clinicians assess the severity of thought disorder.

Q57. Answer: C

Explanation: Clang association refers to speech patterns in which word choice is determined by sound rather than meaning. Words may rhyme or have similar sounds but lack logical connection. The speech may resemble poetry or playful language but becomes disorganized and difficult to follow. This pattern is commonly observed in manic or psychotic states. It reflects disruption in the normal organization of thought. Recognition of this pattern helps clinicians identify underlying mood or psychotic disorders.

Q58. Answer: A

Explanation: Mutism refers to the absence of verbal communication despite the ability to speak. Patients may remain silent even when prompted during interviews. This symptom can occur in severe depression, catatonia, or certain psychotic conditions. The silence may reflect profound emotional distress or psychomotor inhibition. Evaluation should consider both psychiatric and neurological causes. Appropriate treatment depends on identifying the underlying disorder.

Q59. Answer: C

Explanation: Expansive affect refers to exaggerated emotional expression that may appear overly dramatic or theatrical. Individuals may display intense enthusiasm, excitement, or emotional reactions that seem excessive for the situation. This affect pattern is commonly observed in manic episodes. Emotional expression may be loud, animated, and highly expressive. The intensity of emotion often fluctuates rapidly. Observing affect during mental status examination helps identify mood disturbances.

Q60. Answer: C

Explanation: Word salad refers to severely disorganized speech in which words and phrases are combined without logical structure. The resulting language becomes nearly impossible to understand. This pattern reflects profound disturbance in thought organization. It is often observed in advanced stages of psychotic disorders. Communication becomes ineffective because ideas lack coherent connection. Treatment focuses on addressing the underlying psychiatric condition.

Q61. Answer: C

Explanation: Echolalia involves the automatic repetition of words or phrases spoken by another person. The repetition may occur immediately or after a brief delay. This behavior can appear in certain psychiatric and neurological disorders. It reflects impaired control over speech production. The individual may repeat words without understanding or intention. Recognizing echolalia provides insight into disturbances in communication and cognition.

Q62. Answer: C

Explanation: Catastrophic thinking involves expecting the worst possible outcome from a situation. Individuals may interpret minor problems as signs of impending disaster. This cognitive distortion is common in anxiety and depressive disorders. The exaggerated perception of danger increases stress and emotional distress. Over time, catastrophic thinking can reinforce avoidance behaviors. Cognitive therapy techniques often help patients challenge and modify these beliefs.

Q63. Answer: D

Explanation: Delusions of reference involve the belief that ordinary events carry special meaning directed at the individual. Patients may interpret conversations, television programs, or gestures as messages intended specifically for them. These interpretations occur despite lack of objective evidence. Such beliefs reflect distorted perception of environmental stimuli. They are commonly associated with psychotic disorders. Treatment typically focuses on reducing psychotic symptoms.

Q64. Answer: B

Explanation: Conditioning occurs when a neutral stimulus becomes associated with a traumatic or emotionally significant event. After repeated pairing, the stimulus alone can trigger emotional responses. In trauma-related conditions, reminders such as sounds or smells may provoke intense anxiety. The response occurs automatically without conscious intention. This learning process plays a significant role in the development of trauma-related symptoms. Behavioral therapies often focus on gradually reducing these conditioned responses.

Q65. Answer: D

Explanation: Dissociative fugue involves sudden travel away from one's home combined with loss of personal identity. Individuals may appear normal to others but cannot recall important aspects of their past. The condition usually occurs after severe psychological stress or trauma. During the episode the person may adopt a new identity or lifestyle. Memory for the fugue period may remain absent after recovery. Treatment focuses on addressing underlying trauma and restoring personal identity.

Q66. Answer: A

Explanation: Terminal insomnia refers to early morning awakening with inability to fall back asleep. This sleep disturbance is commonly associated with major depressive episodes. Individuals may wake several hours earlier than intended and feel fatigued during the day. The symptom reflects disruption in circadian rhythm and mood regulation. Persistent sleep disturbance can worsen depressive symptoms. Addressing both mood and sleep patterns is important for effective treatment.

Q67. Answer: D

Explanation: Illness anxiety disorder involves excessive fear of having or developing a serious medical condition. Individuals remain preoccupied with health concerns even when medical evaluations show no significant disease. Physical symptoms may be mild or absent, but anxiety about health remains intense. Patients frequently seek reassurance from healthcare providers. The persistent worry can interfere with daily functioning. Treatment typically includes cognitive behavioral therapy aimed at reducing health-related anxiety.

Q68. Answer: B

Explanation: Distractibility refers to difficulty maintaining attention on a single task. Individuals may quickly shift focus from one activity to another. In manic episodes this symptom often leads to multiple unfinished projects or rapidly changing plans. Environmental stimuli easily capture the individual's attention. The inability to maintain concentration interferes with productivity. Treatment aimed at stabilizing mood usually improves attention and focus.

Q69. Answer: C

Explanation: Nihilistic delusions involve beliefs that oneself, others, or the world no longer exist or are ending. Patients may insist that their organs have stopped working or that they are already dead. This belief is strongly fixed and resistant to evidence. Such delusions are most often associated with severe depressive or psychotic disorders. The experience can cause profound emotional distress. Intensive psychiatric treatment is usually required to address these symptoms.

Q70. Answer: D

Explanation: Pressured speech is characterized by rapid, excessive talking that is difficult to interrupt. Individuals may speak loudly and quickly with minimal pauses. This pattern is commonly seen during manic episodes. The person may feel an urgent need to continue speaking without stopping. Rapid speech often accompanies racing thoughts and increased energy. Recognizing this symptom helps clinicians identify mood elevation and potential mania.

Q71. Answer: C

Explanation: Panic attacks involve sudden surges of intense fear or discomfort that reach a peak within minutes. Symptoms often include chest pain, dizziness, trembling, shortness of breath, and fear of losing control. These episodes may occur unexpectedly or in response to triggers. Although the experience can feel life-threatening, it usually resolves within a short period. Recurrent panic attacks may lead to avoidance behaviors. Early recognition allows appropriate psychological and pharmacologic interventions.

Q72. Answer: A

Explanation: Initial insomnia refers to difficulty falling asleep at the beginning of the night. Individuals may lie awake for extended periods despite feeling physically tired. This sleep disturbance is commonly associated with anxiety disorders and certain mood disorders. Persistent difficulty initiating sleep can lead to fatigue and impaired daytime functioning. Stress and racing thoughts often contribute to the problem. Behavioral strategies and treatment of underlying conditions often improve sleep patterns.

Q73. Answer: B

Explanation: Lethargy describes a state of reduced alertness in which a person appears drowsy but can be easily aroused. The individual may respond slowly to questions or stimuli but remains oriented once awake. This level of consciousness may occur due to medication effects, metabolic conditions, or psychiatric illness. Monitoring changes in consciousness is important during clinical assessment. Significant alterations may indicate underlying medical concerns. Appropriate evaluation helps determine the cause and necessary treatment.

Q74. Answer: D

Explanation: Conversion disorder involves neurological symptoms that cannot be explained by medical evaluation. Psychological stress is converted into physical symptoms such as paralysis, blindness, or inability to speak. The symptoms are not intentionally produced. Individuals often appear unaware of the psychological origin of their condition. The disorder represents an unconscious response to overwhelming emotional conflict. Treatment focuses on addressing the psychological stressors contributing to the symptoms.

Q75. Answer: C

Explanation: Factitious disorder involves the intentional production or exaggeration of symptoms to assume the sick role. The primary motivation is psychological rather than external gain. Individuals may fabricate medical histories, alter laboratory samples, or simulate illness. The behavior often leads to repeated hospital visits and unnecessary medical procedures. Unlike malingering, there is no clear external incentive such as financial compensation. Treatment focuses on establishing a therapeutic alliance and addressing underlying psychological needs.

Q76. Answer: A

Explanation: Malingering involves the deliberate fabrication or exaggeration of symptoms for external gain. Common motivations include financial compensation, avoiding work responsibilities, or obtaining medications. Unlike factitious disorder, the individual's goal is practical benefit rather than psychological satisfaction from the sick role. The behavior is considered intentional and conscious. Accurate identification is important to avoid unnecessary medical interventions. Evaluation often requires careful assessment of inconsistencies in reported symptoms.

Q77. Answer: D

Explanation: Obsessive-compulsive personality disorder involves a pervasive pattern of perfectionism, orderliness, and control. Individuals may become so focused on details and rules that they struggle to complete tasks efficiently. Their rigid standards often interfere with flexibility and productivity. Relationships may be affected due to stubbornness and difficulty delegating responsibilities. Unlike obsessive-compulsive disorder, the behaviors are not driven by intrusive thoughts. Psychotherapy helps individuals develop more flexible thinking patterns.

Q78. Answer: A

Explanation: Dependent personality disorder is characterized by excessive reliance on others for emotional and decision-making support. Individuals often feel incapable of functioning independently. They may seek reassurance repeatedly before making even minor choices. Fear of abandonment leads them to tolerate unhealthy relationships. The pattern typically begins in early adulthood and affects many aspects of life. Treatment focuses on building confidence and developing independent decision-making skills.

Q79. Answer: C

Explanation: Avoidant personality disorder involves extreme sensitivity to rejection and criticism. Individuals desire relationships but avoid social interaction due to fear of embarrassment or disapproval. Feelings of inadequacy and low self-esteem often accompany the condition. The avoidance pattern can significantly limit social and occupational opportunities. The behavior differs from social anxiety disorder in that it represents a long-standing personality trait. Psychotherapy focuses on improving self-confidence and interpersonal skills.

Q80. Answer: A

Explanation: Schizoid personality disorder is characterized by detachment from social relationships and limited emotional expression. Individuals typically prefer solitary activities and show little desire for close connections. Emotional responses may appear flat or indifferent. Unlike avoidant personality disorder, the individual does not desire social interaction. The condition often becomes noticeable in early adulthood. Treatment may focus on improving social functioning when the individual seeks help.

Q81. Answer: A

Explanation: Antisocial personality disorder involves a persistent disregard for the rights and safety of others. Individuals often engage in deceitful, manipulative, or aggressive behaviors. They may repeatedly violate social norms or legal boundaries. A lack of remorse for harmful actions is a defining feature of the condition. The disorder typically begins with conduct problems during childhood or adolescence. Treatment is challenging and often focuses on behavioral management and addressing associated conditions.

Q82. Answer: C

Explanation: Paranoid personality disorder involves pervasive distrust and suspicion of others. Individuals often interpret neutral actions as malicious or threatening. They may hold grudges for long periods and remain reluctant to confide in others. The constant suspicion interferes with relationships and daily functioning. Despite their beliefs, they rarely experience the hallucinations or delusions typical of psychotic disorders. Psychotherapy may help individuals develop more balanced interpretations of social situations.

Q83. Answer: A

Explanation: Histrionic personality disorder involves excessive emotionality and a strong desire to be the center of attention. Individuals may behave dramatically or theatrically in social situations. Their emotional expressions often appear exaggerated or shallow. They may become uncomfortable when they are not the focus of attention. Relationships can be superficial and unstable. Psychotherapy helps individuals develop more authentic interpersonal interactions.

Q84. Answer: B

Explanation: Borderline personality disorder is characterized by unstable relationships, emotional instability, and fear of abandonment. Individuals may alternate between viewing others as perfect or completely flawed. Chronic feelings of emptiness and identity disturbance are common. Impulsive behaviors and self-harm may occur during periods of distress. Emotional responses are intense and rapidly changing. Structured psychotherapy programs are considered the most effective treatment.

Q85. Answer: B
Explanation: Hypomania involves a distinct period of elevated or irritable mood lasting at least four days. Symptoms include increased energy, reduced need for sleep, and heightened confidence. Unlike full mania, hypomania does not cause severe impairment or require hospitalization. Individuals may appear unusually productive or sociable. Despite the milder severity, hypomania can still disrupt relationships and judgment. Recognition is important because it often occurs in bipolar II disorder.
Q86. Answer: C
Explanation: Cyclothymic disorder involves chronic fluctuations between hypomanic and mild depressive symptoms. These mood changes persist for at least two years in adults. The symptoms are not severe enough to meet criteria for full manic or major depressive episodes. However, the continuous mood instability can significantly affect daily functioning. Individuals often experience unpredictable emotional shifts. Early recognition may help prevent progression to more severe bipolar disorders.
Q87. Answer: B
Explanation: Anorexia nervosa is characterized by severe restriction of food intake and intense fear of gaining weight. Individuals often maintain body weight significantly below normal levels. Distorted body image leads them to perceive themselves as overweight despite being underweight. The disorder can cause serious medical complications affecting multiple organ systems. Nutritional rehabilitation and psychological therapy are central to treatment. Early intervention improves long-term outcomes.
Q88. Answer: B
Explanation: Bulimia nervosa involves recurrent episodes of binge eating followed by compensatory behaviors. These behaviors may include vomiting, excessive exercise, or misuse of laxatives. Individuals often feel a loss of control during binge episodes. Unlike anorexia nervosa, body weight may remain within a normal range. The cycle of bingeing and purging can lead to significant medical complications. Treatment typically includes psychotherapy and nutritional counseling.
Q89. Answer: B
Explanation: Binge eating disorder involves recurrent episodes of consuming unusually large amounts of food within a short period. Individuals often feel unable to control their eating during these episodes. Unlike bulimia nervosa, compensatory behaviors such as purging are absent. Feelings of guilt or embarrassment frequently follow binge episodes. The disorder can lead to obesity and associated health complications. Treatment commonly includes psychotherapy and behavioral interventions.
Q90. Answer: C
Explanation: Pica is characterized by persistent consumption of nonfood substances. These substances may include dirt, clay, chalk, or paper. The behavior must persist for at least one month and be inappropriate for the individual's developmental level. Nutritional deficiencies and environmental factors may contribute to the condition. Medical complications such as poisoning or intestinal obstruction can occur. Treatment focuses on addressing underlying causes and preventing harmful ingestion.
Q91. Answer: A
Explanation: Rumination disorder involves repeated regurgitation of food after eating. The regurgitated food may be re-chewed, swallowed again, or spit out. The behavior occurs without nausea or gastrointestinal illness. It can appear in infants, children, or adults. The disorder may lead to nutritional deficiencies and weight loss. Behavioral therapy is often effective in reducing the behavior.
Q92. Answer: C
Explanation: Avoidant restrictive food intake disorder involves limited food consumption that leads to nutritional deficiency or weight loss. The restriction is not related to concerns about body weight or shape. Individuals may avoid food due to sensory sensitivity, fear of choking, or lack of interest in eating. The disorder can occur across all age groups. Nutritional deficiencies and growth problems may develop if untreated. Treatment focuses on nutritional rehabilitation and behavioral therapy.
Q93. Answer: C

Explanation: Somnambulism, also known as sleepwalking, occurs during deep stages of non-REM sleep. Individuals may sit up, walk around, or perform activities while remaining partially asleep. Episodes usually occur during the first third of the night. Memory of the event is often absent upon waking. Stress, sleep deprivation, and certain medications may increase the likelihood of episodes. Ensuring a safe sleeping environment is an important management strategy.

Q94. Answer: B

Explanation: Narcolepsy is a neurological disorder characterized by excessive daytime sleepiness. Individuals may suddenly fall asleep during normal daily activities. These episodes can occur even after adequate nighttime sleep. Additional symptoms may include sudden muscle weakness triggered by emotions and vivid dream experiences. The condition results from abnormal regulation of sleep-wake cycles. Treatment often involves medications and behavioral strategies to manage symptoms.

Q95. Answer: D

Explanation: Obstructive sleep apnea involves repeated episodes of airway obstruction during sleep. Breathing pauses may last several seconds and occur many times each night. Loud snoring and daytime fatigue are common symptoms. The condition reduces oxygen levels and disrupts normal sleep cycles. Untreated sleep apnea increases risk of cardiovascular disease and other health problems. Treatment may include lifestyle changes, medical devices, or surgical intervention.

Q96. Answer: C

Explanation: Sleep terror disorder involves sudden episodes of intense fear during sleep. The individual may scream, appear frightened, and show signs of autonomic arousal. Episodes usually occur during deep non-REM sleep and often happen in children. Attempts to comfort the individual may be unsuccessful because they remain partially asleep. Memory of the event is typically absent after waking. The condition often resolves naturally as the child grows older.

Q97. Answer: B

Explanation: Nightmare disorder involves recurrent vivid dreams that are frightening or disturbing. These dreams occur during REM sleep and usually awaken the individual. After waking, the person is alert and able to recall the dream in detail. The distress associated with the dreams can interfere with sleep quality. Stress, trauma, or certain medications may increase occurrence. Treatment often focuses on stress reduction and sleep hygiene strategies.

Q98. Answer: C

Explanation: Sleep paralysis occurs when the body remains temporarily paralyzed during the transition between sleep and wakefulness. Individuals may feel awake but unable to move or speak. Episodes typically last a few seconds to minutes. Although the experience can be frightening, it is usually harmless. Sleep deprivation and irregular sleep schedules can increase the likelihood of episodes. Improving sleep habits often reduces frequency.

Q99. Answer: D

Explanation: Circadian rhythm sleep disorders occur when the body's internal clock becomes misaligned with external schedules. Shift work is a common cause because sleep occurs during times when the body expects wakefulness. Individuals may struggle to fall asleep during the day and feel fatigued during work hours. Chronic misalignment can impair concentration and mood. Adjusting light exposure and sleep schedules may improve symptoms. Some individuals benefit from structured sleep routines or medical guidance.

Q100. Answer: A

Explanation: Insomnia disorder involves ongoing difficulty with sleep initiation, maintenance, or quality. Individuals often feel unrefreshed after sleep and experience daytime fatigue or impaired concentration. The condition may occur independently or alongside other medical or psychiatric disorders. Stress, poor sleep habits, and mood disturbances frequently contribute to insomnia. Chronic sleep disruption can affect cognitive performance and emotional well-being. Treatment commonly includes behavioral interventions and addressing underlying contributing factors.

Question (101-200)

Q101. A patient with major depressive disorder reports persistent sadness, loss of interest in activities, and early morning awakening for the past two months despite adherence to medication. What is the most appropriate next step in management?

(A) Reevaluate treatment response and consider medication adjustment

(B) Ignore symptoms if the patient appears stable

(C) Continue the same medication without reassessment

(D) Immediately discontinue all antidepressant medications

Q102. A patient experiencing acute panic attacks reports palpitations, sweating, and fear of losing control. Which intervention is most helpful during the acute episode?

(A) Instruct the patient to avoid discussing the symptoms

(B) Encourage slow breathing and grounding techniques

(C) Ignore the symptoms as they are harmless

(D) Recommend isolation until symptoms subside

Q103. A patient receiving lithium therapy reports nausea, tremor, and excessive thirst. Which action should the clinician take first?

(A) Assess lithium serum level

(B) Discontinue treatment immediately without evaluation

(C) Ignore symptoms if mild

(D) Increase lithium dose

Q104. A patient diagnosed with schizophrenia begins hearing voices that command harmful actions. What is the priority clinical intervention?

(A) Delay evaluation until next appointment

(B) Assess safety risk and initiate appropriate intervention

(C) Ignore the hallucinations

(D) Encourage the patient to obey the voices

Q105. A patient with bipolar disorder presents with elevated mood, decreased need for sleep, and excessive spending. Which condition is most consistent with these symptoms?

(A) Panic disorder

(B) Manic episode

(C) Major depressive episode

(D) Adjustment disorder

Q106. A patient with generalized anxiety disorder reports constant worry about daily activities. Which therapeutic approach is most effective long-term?

(A) Sedation without psychotherapy

(B) Avoid discussing anxiety triggers

(C) Ignore symptoms

(D) Cognitive behavioral therapy

Q107. A patient treated with antipsychotic medication develops muscle rigidity and high fever. Which condition should be suspected?

(A) Panic disorder

(B) Generalized anxiety disorder

(C) Serotonin syndrome

(D) Neuroleptic malignant syndrome

Q108. A patient expresses persistent feelings of worthlessness and guilt following job loss. Which nursing intervention is most therapeutic?

(A) Dismiss the patient's concerns as temporary

(B) Encourage expression of feelings in a supportive environment
(C) Encourage isolation
(D) Change the topic during discussion

Q109. A patient with alcohol use disorder develops tremors and agitation after stopping alcohol consumption. What condition is likely occurring?
(A) Social anxiety disorder
(B) Major depressive disorder
(C) Alcohol withdrawal syndrome
(D) Bipolar mania

Q110. A patient reports difficulty concentrating, irritability, and fatigue after exposure to prolonged stress at work. Which diagnosis is most consistent?
(A) Bipolar disorder
(B) Panic disorder
(C) Schizophrenia
(D) Adjustment disorder

Q111. A patient receiving antidepressant therapy reports improvement in mood but persistent insomnia. What is the most appropriate next step?
(A) Increase dose without assessment
(B) Ignore sleep issues
(C) Stop antidepressant therapy immediately
(D) Evaluate sleep hygiene and medication timing

Q112. A patient expresses fear of leaving home due to worry about having panic attacks in public. Which disorder is most likely present?
(A) Major depression
(B) Agoraphobia
(C) Schizoaffective disorder
(D) Bipolar disorder

Q113. A patient treated with selective serotonin reuptake inhibitors reports nausea during the first week of therapy. What is the most appropriate clinical response?
(A) Educate that mild gastrointestinal symptoms may occur initially
(B) Double the medication dose
(C) Stop treatment immediately
(D) Ignore patient concerns

Q114. A patient experiencing severe depression expresses thoughts about death but denies a specific plan. What is the priority assessment?
(A) Ignore the statement
(B) Discharge the patient immediately
(C) Change the subject
(D) Evaluate suicide risk and protective factors

Q115. A patient diagnosed with obsessive compulsive disorder reports repetitive hand washing due to fear of contamination. What is the primary goal of therapy?
(A) Encourage compulsions
(B) Reinforce avoidance
(C) Reduce compulsive behaviors and anxiety
(D) Ignore the behavior

Q116. A patient with schizophrenia demonstrates flat affect and limited speech. These symptoms represent which category?
(A) Positive symptoms

(B) Mood symptoms
(C) Cognitive symptoms
(D) Negative symptoms

Q117. A patient reports feeling excessively energetic and engaging in multiple projects without completion. Which clinical condition is most likely?

(A) Social anxiety
(B) Adjustment disorder
(C) Mania
(D) Depression

Q118. A patient undergoing psychotherapy expresses anger toward the therapist during sessions. How should the clinician respond?

(A) Ignore the statement
(B) Explore the feelings within the therapeutic relationship
(C) Terminate therapy immediately
(D) Avoid discussing emotions

Q119. A patient with chronic anxiety reports muscle tension, restlessness, and difficulty sleeping. Which disorder best matches these symptoms?

(A) Dissociative disorder
(B) Generalized anxiety disorder
(C) Bipolar disorder
(D) Schizophrenia

Q120. A patient expresses feelings of emptiness and unstable relationships with intense fear of abandonment. Which personality disorder is suggested?

(A) Narcissistic personality disorder
(B) Borderline personality disorder
(C) Avoidant personality disorder
(D) Obsessive personality disorder

Q121. A patient who recently survived a traumatic accident reports intrusive memories, nightmares, and avoidance of reminders related to the event for several weeks. Which disorder is most consistent with these symptoms?

(A) Social anxiety disorder
(B) Post-traumatic stress disorder
(C) Generalized anxiety disorder
(D) Bipolar disorder

Q122. A patient being treated with antipsychotic medication begins experiencing involuntary lip smacking and tongue movements. What condition should be suspected?

(A) Acute anxiety reaction
(B) Tardive dyskinesia
(C) Panic disorder
(D) Serotonin syndrome

Q123. A patient reports persistent fear of social interactions and worries about being judged negatively by others. Which disorder best explains this presentation?

(A) Dissociative identity disorder
(B) Social anxiety disorder
(C) Schizophrenia
(D) Bipolar disorder

Q124. A patient diagnosed with depression reports difficulty making decisions and decreased ability to focus on daily tasks. Which symptom category does this represent?

(A) Psychotic symptom
(B) Behavioral symptom
(C) Cognitive symptom
(D) Somatic symptom

Q125. A patient presents with extreme mood swings, alternating between emotional highs and severe lows over several months. Which condition should be considered?
(A) Obsessive compulsive disorder
(B) Panic disorder
(C) Adjustment disorder
(D) Bipolar disorder

Q126. A patient reports hearing voices commenting on daily actions while alone. Which symptom type is being described?
(A) Illusion
(B) Auditory hallucination
(C) Obsession
(D) Delusion

Q127. A patient frequently checks locks and appliances multiple times before leaving home due to persistent worry something bad will occur. Which disorder best explains this behavior?
(A) Obsessive compulsive disorder
(B) Dissociative disorder
(C) Schizoaffective disorder
(D) Bipolar disorder

Q128. A patient with schizophrenia displays reduced emotional expression and minimal motivation to engage in daily activities. Which symptom classification applies?
(A) Anxiety symptom
(B) Positive symptom
(C) Negative symptom
(D) Mood symptom

Q129. A patient experiencing intense fear when speaking in front of groups avoids presentations at work. Which treatment strategy is commonly effective?
(A) Gradual exposure therapy
(B) Ignoring the fear response
(C) Encouraging avoidance
(D) Immediate medication discontinuation

Q130. A patient reports sudden episodes of intense fear accompanied by shortness of breath, dizziness, and chest discomfort. What condition should be suspected?
(A) Bipolar disorder
(B) Major depressive disorder
(C) Schizophrenia
(D) Panic disorder

Q131. A patient reports chronic feelings of hopelessness and lack of motivation lasting more than two years. Which diagnosis is most consistent?
(A) Dissociative disorder
(B) Persistent depressive disorder
(C) Bipolar disorder
(D) Panic disorder

Q132. A patient with severe anxiety complains of constant muscle tension and restlessness throughout the day. Which disorder is most likely?

(A) Delusional disorder
(B) Bipolar disorder
(C) Generalized anxiety disorder
(D) Schizophrenia

Q133. A patient expresses belief that strangers on television are sending personal messages through broadcasts. What symptom is represented?
(A) Hallucination
(B) Phobia
(C) Delusion of reference
(D) Obsession

Q134. A patient experiencing severe depressive symptoms reports loss of pleasure in previously enjoyable activities. What term describes this symptom?
(A) Compulsion
(B) Mania
(C) Anhedonia
(D) Hallucination

Q135. A patient who frequently exaggerates achievements and seeks constant admiration may exhibit traits of which personality disorder?
(A) Borderline personality disorder
(B) Avoidant personality disorder
(C) Dependent personality disorder
(D) Narcissistic personality disorder

Q136. A patient describes sudden inability to recall important personal information after a stressful event. Which condition is most consistent with this symptom?
(A) Social anxiety disorder
(B) Bipolar disorder
(C) Dissociative amnesia
(D) Panic disorder

Q137. A patient reports excessive concern about physical health despite repeated normal medical evaluations. Which disorder should be considered?
(A) Schizoaffective disorder
(B) Panic disorder
(C) Illness anxiety disorder
(D) Bipolar disorder

Q138. A patient becomes extremely distressed when separated from a close family member. Which disorder is commonly associated with this symptom in children?
(A) Conduct disorder
(B) Schizophrenia
(C) Separation anxiety disorder
(D) Bipolar disorder

Q139. A patient exhibits persistent patterns of disregard for the rights of others and engages in manipulative behavior. Which personality disorder is suggested?
(A) Dependent personality disorder
(B) Obsessive personality disorder
(C) Avoidant personality disorder
(D) Antisocial personality disorder

Q140. A patient reports recurrent thoughts about harming others but has no intention to act on them. These thoughts cause significant distress. What symptom is present?

(A) Hallucination
(B) Phobia
(C) Obsession
(D) Delusion

Q141. A patient avoids crowded places because of fear that escape may be difficult during a panic episode. Which condition is most likely present?
(A) Bipolar disorder
(B) Agoraphobia
(C) Schizophrenia
(D) Dissociative disorder

Q142. A patient receiving antidepressant therapy begins experiencing increased energy and decreased need for sleep. What should be considered?
(A) Treatment success without concern
(B) Immediate medication discontinuation without assessment
(C) Normal response requiring no evaluation
(D) Possible manic switch

Q143. A patient frequently seeks reassurance from others and struggles to make decisions independently. Which personality disorder may be present?
(A) Narcissistic personality disorder
(B) Dependent personality disorder
(C) Schizotypal personality disorder
(D) Antisocial personality disorder

Q144. A patient experiences persistent sadness, fatigue, and reduced appetite lasting several weeks. Which diagnosis is most consistent?
(A) Panic disorder
(B) Delusional disorder
(C) Schizophrenia
(D) Major depressive disorder

Q145. A patient reports repeated episodes of intense anger and impulsive behavior that strain relationships. Which disorder may be associated with these features?
(A) Avoidant personality disorder
(B) Obsessive personality disorder
(C) Dependent personality disorder
(D) Borderline personality disorder

Q146. A patient complains of persistent difficulty falling asleep despite feeling exhausted. Which condition best describes this problem?
(A) Panic disorder
(B) Insomnia disorder
(C) Bipolar disorder
(D) Schizoaffective disorder

Q147. A patient reports sudden episodes of overwhelming fear accompanied by trembling and sweating that peak within minutes. What condition should be suspected?
(A) Dissociative disorder
(B) Schizophrenia
(C) Major depression
(D) Panic attack

Q148. A patient displays exaggerated emotional expression and constantly seeks attention from others. Which personality disorder may be indicated?

(A) Histrionic personality disorder
(B) Avoidant personality disorder
(C) Schizoid personality disorder
(D) Dependent personality disorder

Q149. A patient believes coworkers are secretly plotting against them despite lack of evidence. Which symptom type does this represent?
(A) Compulsion
(B) Hallucination
(C) Obsession
(D) Paranoid delusion

Q150. A patient reports persistent fatigue, poor concentration, and feelings of hopelessness for several months. Which mental health condition should be considered?
(A) Depressive disorder
(B) Bipolar mania
(C) Panic disorder
(D) Dissociative disorder

Q151. A patient reports persistent feelings of tension, irritability, and difficulty concentrating for several months without a specific trigger. Which disorder is most consistent with this presentation?
(A) Generalized anxiety disorder
(B) Bipolar disorder
(C) Dissociative disorder
(D) Schizoaffective disorder

Q152. A patient suddenly becomes confused, disoriented, and experiences fluctuating levels of consciousness while hospitalized. What condition should be suspected?
(A) Panic disorder
(B) Personality disorder
(C) Delirium
(D) Major depression

Q153. A patient with schizophrenia reports hearing voices arguing with each other. What symptom category does this represent?
(A) Delusion
(B) Obsession
(C) Auditory hallucination
(D) Compulsion

Q154. A patient frequently exaggerates personal achievements and believes they are superior to others. Which personality disorder is most consistent with this pattern?
(A) Schizoid personality disorder
(B) Dependent personality disorder
(C) Narcissistic personality disorder
(D) Avoidant personality disorder

Q155. A patient experiences sudden memory loss about personal identity after witnessing a traumatic event. Which disorder should be considered?
(A) Panic disorder
(B) Bipolar disorder
(C) Delusional disorder
(D) Dissociative amnesia

Q156. A patient avoids social interactions due to intense fear of embarrassment and criticism. Which disorder is most likely present?

(A) Bipolar disorder
(B) Panic disorder
(C) Schizophrenia
(D) Social anxiety disorder

Q157. A patient repeatedly arranges items symmetrically on a desk to relieve anxiety caused by intrusive thoughts. Which disorder best explains this behavior?
(A) Dissociative disorder
(B) Obsessive compulsive disorder
(C) Bipolar disorder
(D) Panic disorder

Q158. A patient reports excessive daytime sleepiness and frequent unintended sleep episodes during daily activities. Which disorder should be suspected?
(A) Panic disorder
(B) Major depression
(C) Schizophrenia
(D) Narcolepsy

Q159. A patient persistently believes that a spouse is unfaithful despite lack of evidence. Which symptom category does this represent?
(A) Hallucination
(B) Compulsion
(C) Delusion
(D) Obsession

Q160. A patient complains of repeated headaches and stomach pain but medical tests reveal no physical cause. Which disorder should be considered?
(A) Schizophrenia
(B) Panic disorder
(C) Bipolar disorder
(D) Somatic symptom disorder

Q161. A patient demonstrates extreme emotional detachment and prefers solitary activities. Which personality disorder may be indicated?
(A) Dependent personality disorder
(B) Schizoid personality disorder
(C) Narcissistic personality disorder
(D) Borderline personality disorder

Q162. A patient experiences intrusive memories and heightened startle response after surviving a natural disaster. Which condition should be considered?
(A) Dissociative disorder
(B) Panic disorder
(C) Post-traumatic stress disorder
(D) Bipolar disorder

Q163. A patient repeatedly washes hands due to fear of contamination despite knowing the fear is irrational. What symptom type is being demonstrated?
(A) Phobia
(B) Hallucination
(C) Delusion
(D) Compulsion

Q164. A patient reports episodes of sudden sadness and crying that occur without a clear reason. Which condition may be present?

(A) Schizophrenia
(B) Depressive disorder
(C) Bipolar mania
(D) Panic disorder

Q165. A patient constantly fears being criticized or rejected and therefore avoids forming close relationships. Which personality disorder is most consistent with this pattern?
(A) Antisocial personality disorder
(B) Histrionic personality disorder
(C) Narcissistic personality disorder
(D) Avoidant personality disorder

Q166. A patient displays inflated self-esteem, increased talkativeness, and decreased need for sleep. Which mood state does this represent?
(A) Anxiety
(B) Depression
(C) Dissociation
(D) Mania

Q167. A patient experiences persistent fatigue, low mood, and loss of interest lasting several weeks. Which condition is most likely present?
(A) Major depressive disorder
(B) Delusional disorder
(C) Schizophrenia
(D) Panic disorder

Q168. A patient frequently lies and manipulates others for personal gain without remorse. Which personality disorder may be indicated?
(A) Schizoid personality disorder
(B) Dependent personality disorder
(C) Antisocial personality disorder
(D) Avoidant personality disorder

Q169. A patient develops sudden confusion and agitation after starting a new medication. Which condition should be evaluated?
(A) Panic disorder
(B) Bipolar disorder
(C) Delirium
(D) Depression

Q170. A patient expresses excessive pride and emotional expression that appears theatrical during conversations. Which personality disorder may be suggested?
(A) Dependent personality disorder
(B) Avoidant personality disorder
(C) Schizoid personality disorder
(D) Histrionic personality disorder

Q171. A patient believes that strangers are constantly observing and judging them. Which symptom is being described?
(A) Obsession
(B) Paranoid delusion
(C) Compulsion
(D) Hallucination

Q172. A patient complains of repeated intrusive thoughts about contamination that cause severe anxiety. What symptom type is present?

(A) Obsession
(B) Phobia
(C) Hallucination
(D) Delusion

Q173. A patient reports extreme fear of heights and avoids tall buildings or bridges. Which disorder is most consistent with this symptom?
(A) Dissociative disorder
(B) Specific phobia
(C) Schizophrenia
(D) Bipolar disorder

Q174. A patient displays persistent sadness along with changes in appetite and sleep patterns. Which condition should be considered?
(A) Panic disorder
(B) Delusional disorder
(C) Schizophrenia
(D) Depressive disorder

Q175. A patient avoids speaking in meetings due to fear of humiliation. Which condition is most likely present?
(A) Bipolar disorder
(B) Dissociative disorder
(C) Social anxiety disorder
(D) Panic disorder

Q176. A patient with bipolar disorder reports rapid mood shifts occurring within a single day. Which pattern may be occurring?
(A) Panic disorder
(B) Rapid cycling mood pattern
(C) Chronic depression
(D) Dissociative disorder

Q177. A patient persistently believes they possess extraordinary abilities and deserve special recognition. Which personality disorder is suggested?
(A) Avoidant personality disorder
(B) Schizoid personality disorder
(C) Dependent personality disorder
(D) Narcissistic personality disorder

Q178. A patient experiences sudden episodes of fear with heart palpitations and dizziness. Which condition should be suspected?
(A) Schizophrenia
(B) Panic attack
(C) Dissociative disorder
(D) Major depression

Q179. A patient complains of constant worry about multiple aspects of life such as finances, health, and family responsibilities. Which disorder is most consistent with these symptoms?
(A) Bipolar disorder
(B) Schizophrenia
(C) Delusional disorder
(D) Generalized anxiety disorder

Q180. A patient describes feeling emotionally empty and fears abandonment in relationships. Which personality disorder may be present?

(A) Avoidant personality disorder
(B) Borderline personality disorder
(C) Narcissistic personality disorder
(D) Schizoid personality disorder

Q181. A patient reports repetitive behaviors such as counting steps while walking to reduce anxiety. Which disorder best explains this behavior?

(A) Panic disorder
(B) Bipolar disorder
(C) Obsessive compulsive disorder
(D) Schizophrenia

Q182. A patient persistently complains about physical symptoms but medical examinations reveal no underlying disease. Which condition may be indicated?

(A) Panic disorder
(B) Somatic symptom disorder
(C) Bipolar disorder
(D) Schizophrenia

Q183. A patient experiences difficulty remembering personal information after a traumatic event. Which disorder is most consistent with this symptom?

(A) Social anxiety disorder
(B) Bipolar disorder
(C) Dissociative amnesia
(D) Panic disorder

Q184. A patient avoids interacting with coworkers due to fear of being judged or criticized. Which disorder should be considered?

(A) Schizophrenia
(B) Delusional disorder
(C) Social anxiety disorder
(D) Bipolar disorder

Q185. A patient with depression reports inability to experience pleasure in previously enjoyable activities. Which symptom is this?

(A) Mania
(B) Anhedonia
(C) Delusion
(D) Hallucination

Q186. A patient displays persistent distrust and suspicion toward others without sufficient reason. Which personality disorder may be present?

(A) Dependent personality disorder
(B) Histrionic personality disorder
(C) Avoidant personality disorder
(D) Paranoid personality disorder

Q187. A patient experiences extreme emotional reactions and unstable interpersonal relationships. Which personality disorder is suggested?

(A) Schizoid personality disorder
(B) Narcissistic personality disorder
(C) Avoidant personality disorder
(D) Borderline personality disorder

Q188. A patient demonstrates excessive emotionality and dramatic speech to gain attention. Which personality disorder may be indicated?

(A) Antisocial personality disorder
(B) Dependent personality disorder
(C) Schizoid personality disorder
(D) Histrionic personality disorder

Q189. A patient constantly relies on others to make everyday decisions and fears being alone. Which personality disorder may be present?
(A) Antisocial personality disorder
(B) Dependent personality disorder
(C) Narcissistic personality disorder
(D) Paranoid personality disorder

Q190. A patient experiences recurring intrusive thoughts about harming someone but feels distressed by the thoughts. What symptom type is present?
(A) Delusion
(B) Phobia
(C) Hallucination
(D) Obsession

Q191. A patient reports persistent fatigue and reduced energy even after adequate sleep. Which condition may be present?
(A) Dissociative disorder
(B) Panic disorder
(C) Depressive disorder
(D) Schizophrenia

Q192. A patient displays sudden confusion and disorganized thinking during hospitalization for infection. Which condition should be suspected?
(A) Delirium
(B) Bipolar disorder
(C) Panic disorder
(D) Personality disorder

Q193. A patient believes neighbors are secretly recording conversations inside the house. Which symptom type is being described?
(A) Phobia
(B) Hallucination
(C) Delusion
(D) Obsession

Q194. A patient experiences excessive worry about developing serious illness despite normal medical results. Which disorder should be considered?
(A) Illness anxiety disorder
(B) Panic disorder
(C) Bipolar disorder
(D) Schizophrenia

Q195. A patient suddenly becomes fearful when entering elevators and avoids them whenever possible. Which condition is most consistent with this behavior?
(A) Schizophrenia
(B) Bipolar disorder
(C) Specific phobia
(D) Dissociative disorder

Q196. A patient reports difficulty maintaining attention and frequently becomes distracted during conversations. Which symptom category is this?

(A) Compulsion
(B) Hallucination
(C) Delusion
(D) Cognitive symptom

Q197. A patient expresses feelings of worthlessness and guilt for minor mistakes. Which mental health condition should be considered?

(A) Panic disorder
(B) Schizophrenia
(C) Bipolar mania
(D) Major depressive disorder

Q198. A patient reports extreme fear of traveling alone due to concern about experiencing panic symptoms. Which condition may be present?

(A) Agoraphobia
(B) Dissociative disorder
(C) Bipolar disorder
(D) Schizophrenia

Q199. A patient demonstrates persistent emotional coldness and limited interest in social relationships. Which personality disorder may be indicated?

(A) Histrionic personality disorder
(B) Borderline personality disorder
(C) Narcissistic personality disorder
(D) Schizoid personality disorder

Q200. A patient reports continuous worry, muscle tension, and difficulty relaxing for several months. Which disorder is most consistent with these symptoms?

(A) Dissociative disorder
(B) Bipolar disorder
(C) Schizophrenia
(D) Generalized anxiety disorder

Answer Key and Explanation (101-200)

Q101. Answer: A

Explanation: When a patient continues to experience depressive symptoms despite treatment, reassessment of treatment effectiveness is necessary. Clinicians evaluate symptom persistence, medication adherence, and possible need for dosage change or alternative therapy. Treatment-resistant symptoms often require medication adjustment or addition of psychotherapy. Regular monitoring helps prevent worsening depression and improves patient outcomes. Early intervention after inadequate response helps reduce functional impairment and enhances recovery.

Q102. Answer: B

Explanation: Panic attacks involve intense autonomic arousal and fear that can escalate rapidly. Teaching controlled breathing and grounding techniques helps regulate the autonomic nervous system. These strategies reduce hyperventilation and restore a sense of control. Calm reassurance from the clinician also supports emotional stabilization. Behavioral techniques during an episode are effective in preventing escalation of panic symptoms.

Q103. Answer: A

Explanation: Lithium has a narrow therapeutic index, making serum level monitoring essential. Symptoms such as tremor, nausea, and thirst may indicate toxicity or high serum concentration. Immediate laboratory evaluation helps determine whether dosage adjustment is necessary. Early detection prevents progression to severe toxicity affecting neurological and renal systems. Regular monitoring ensures safe and effective therapy.

Q104. Answer: B

Explanation: Command hallucinations can pose serious safety risks for both the patient and others. Immediate assessment determines the level of danger and necessary protective measures. Clinicians must evaluate intent, impulse control, and ability to resist the hallucinated commands. Rapid intervention may include hospitalization, medication adjustment, or crisis management. Ensuring safety remains the primary priority in such situations.

Q105. Answer: B

Explanation: Mania is characterized by elevated or irritable mood accompanied by increased activity or energy. Symptoms often include decreased need for sleep, impulsive behavior, and inflated self-esteem. Risky behaviors such as excessive spending are commonly observed. Identification of mania is essential because it requires specific pharmacologic treatment such as mood stabilizers. Early recognition prevents harmful consequences and functional impairment.

Q106. Answer: D

Explanation: Cognitive behavioral therapy helps patients recognize and modify maladaptive thought patterns that contribute to anxiety. The therapy teaches coping strategies and behavioral techniques that reduce excessive worry. Over time, patients develop skills to manage stress and challenge irrational fears. Research consistently demonstrates strong long-term outcomes with this structured therapy. Combining CBT with medication may further improve symptom control.

Q107. Answer: D

Explanation: Neuroleptic malignant syndrome is a rare but life-threatening reaction associated with antipsychotic medications. It is characterized by hyperthermia, muscle rigidity, altered mental status, and autonomic instability. Immediate medical evaluation is essential because the condition can rapidly worsen. Early recognition allows prompt discontinuation of the offending medication and initiation of supportive treatment. Delay in management significantly increases morbidity and mortality.

Q108. Answer: B

Explanation: Therapeutic communication allows patients to express emotional distress without judgment. Encouraging discussion helps individuals process feelings and gain insight into their experiences. A supportive environment strengthens the therapeutic alliance and reduces feelings of isolation. Emotional validation improves coping ability and psychological resilience. Effective communication is fundamental in psychiatric care.

Q109. Answer: C

Explanation: Alcohol withdrawal occurs when a person who is dependent on alcohol abruptly stops or reduces intake. Symptoms typically include tremors, agitation, anxiety, and autonomic instability. Severe cases may progress to seizures or delirium tremens. Early recognition allows initiation of medical management to prevent complications. Monitoring and supportive treatment are critical during the withdrawal period.

Q110. Answer: D

Explanation: Adjustment disorder occurs when emotional or behavioral symptoms develop in response to identifiable stressors. Symptoms typically arise within a few months of the stress event. Individuals often experience anxiety, depressed mood, or difficulty functioning. Treatment focuses on coping strategies, stress management, and supportive therapy. Early intervention can prevent progression to more severe mental health conditions.

Q111. Answer: D

Explanation: Sleep disturbances may persist even when depressive symptoms improve. Assessment of sleep hygiene practices and medication timing helps identify contributing factors. Adjusting medication schedule or incorporating behavioral strategies may improve sleep quality. Addressing insomnia is important because poor sleep can worsen mental health symptoms. Comprehensive evaluation ensures balanced treatment outcomes.

Q112. Answer: B

Explanation: Agoraphobia involves intense fear of situations where escape may be difficult or help unavailable during panic symptoms. Individuals often avoid public places or crowded environments. The condition frequently develops alongside panic disorder. Avoidance behaviors can significantly impair daily functioning. Treatment typically includes psychotherapy and gradual exposure to feared situations.

Q113. Answer: A

Explanation: Gastrointestinal discomfort is a common early side effect of many antidepressant medications. Symptoms often resolve as the body adjusts to the medication. Providing education helps patients understand the temporary nature of the effect. Reassurance improves adherence and reduces unnecessary discontinuation. Monitoring ensures that symptoms do not worsen or persist.

Q114. Answer: D

Explanation: Any mention of death or suicidal thoughts requires careful evaluation. Clinicians assess intent, planning, protective factors, and support systems. Early risk assessment allows implementation of safety planning and intervention. Even passive thoughts can indicate significant distress. Thorough assessment ensures timely prevention of potential self-harm.

Q115. Answer: C

Explanation: Obsessive compulsive disorder involves intrusive thoughts and repetitive behaviors performed to reduce anxiety. Effective treatment focuses on reducing the compulsive rituals and addressing underlying fears. Cognitive behavioral strategies help individuals resist compulsions and tolerate anxiety. Over time, patients learn that feared consequences do not occur. Gradual reduction of compulsive behaviors improves functioning and quality of life.

Q116. Answer: D

Explanation: Negative symptoms involve diminished emotional expression and reduced motivation. Individuals may display limited speech, social withdrawal, and decreased facial expression. These symptoms differ from positive symptoms such as hallucinations or delusions. Negative symptoms often contribute to long-term functional impairment. Recognition helps guide comprehensive treatment planning.

Q117. Answer: C
Explanation: Mania is characterized by increased energy, decreased need for sleep, and heightened goal-directed activity. Individuals may start numerous tasks but fail to complete them due to distractibility. Risk-taking behaviors and impulsive decisions frequently accompany these symptoms. Early identification is crucial because untreated mania can lead to serious consequences. Mood stabilizing treatment helps restore emotional balance.
Q118. Answer: B
Explanation: Emotional reactions toward the therapist may represent important therapeutic material. Exploring these feelings can provide insight into interpersonal patterns. Addressing emotions within therapy strengthens trust and promotes self-awareness. The therapeutic alliance allows safe discussion of difficult experiences. Constructive exploration enhances treatment progress.
Q119. Answer: B
Explanation: Generalized anxiety disorder involves persistent and excessive worry about various aspects of daily life. Physical symptoms such as muscle tension and sleep disturbance frequently accompany the condition. The anxiety is typically difficult to control and occurs for extended periods. Early treatment helps reduce psychological distress and improve functioning. Both therapy and medication may be beneficial.
Q120. Answer: B
Explanation: Borderline personality disorder involves instability in relationships, self-image, and emotional regulation. Individuals often fear abandonment and experience intense mood shifts. Interpersonal conflicts and impulsive behaviors are common. Early diagnosis supports structured therapy approaches that improve emotional stability. Psychotherapy remains the primary treatment strategy.
Q121. Answer: B
Explanation: Post-traumatic stress disorder develops after exposure to a traumatic event and is characterized by intrusive memories, nightmares, and heightened psychological distress when reminded of the trauma. Individuals often attempt to avoid places, conversations, or situations associated with the event. Hyperarousal symptoms such as irritability and sleep disturbance may also occur. The condition can significantly interfere with social and occupational functioning. Early identification and treatment improve recovery and help prevent long-term psychological complications.
Q122. Answer: B
Explanation: Tardive dyskinesia is a movement disorder associated with long-term use of certain antipsychotic medications. It is characterized by repetitive, involuntary movements often affecting the face, lips, and tongue. These movements may become persistent and can worsen if not addressed early. Regular monitoring during antipsychotic treatment is essential for early detection. Prompt evaluation allows clinicians to modify therapy and reduce the risk of permanent symptoms.
Q123. Answer: B
Explanation: Social anxiety disorder involves intense fear of social situations where individuals may feel scrutinized or judged. People with this condition often avoid gatherings, presentations, or conversations with unfamiliar individuals. The fear can cause significant distress and impair academic, occupational, or interpersonal functioning. Physical symptoms such as sweating or trembling may occur during exposure to feared situations. Evidence-based treatments include psychotherapy and pharmacologic interventions.
Q124. Answer: C
Explanation: Cognitive symptoms of depression include impaired concentration, indecisiveness, and slowed thinking. These difficulties can affect work performance, academic tasks, and daily functioning. The cognitive component of depression is often overlooked but contributes significantly to disability. Treatment targeting mood improvement frequently leads to cognitive recovery as well. Early recognition helps guide comprehensive treatment planning.
Q125. Answer: D

Explanation: Bipolar disorder is characterized by episodes of mania or hypomania alternating with episodes of depression. Mood shifts may involve periods of high energy, reduced sleep, and increased activity followed by periods of sadness and fatigue. These fluctuations can disrupt relationships and occupational functioning. Accurate diagnosis is critical because treatment differs significantly from unipolar depression. Mood stabilizing medications are commonly used in management.

Q126. Answer: B

Explanation: Auditory hallucinations involve hearing sounds or voices without an external stimulus. They are commonly associated with psychotic disorders such as schizophrenia. Individuals may perceive voices commenting on behavior or giving instructions. These experiences can be distressing and interfere with normal functioning. Assessment and appropriate pharmacologic treatment help reduce symptom severity.

Q127. Answer: A

Explanation: Obsessive compulsive disorder is characterized by intrusive thoughts and repetitive behaviors performed to relieve anxiety. Compulsive checking is a common manifestation of the disorder. Individuals feel driven to perform rituals despite recognizing that the behavior is excessive. These repetitive actions can consume significant time and disrupt daily activities. Behavioral therapy and medication often improve symptom control.

Q128. Answer: C

Explanation: Negative symptoms represent a reduction or absence of normal emotional and behavioral functions. Examples include diminished facial expression, lack of motivation, and social withdrawal. These symptoms can significantly impair daily functioning and quality of life. They often persist even when positive symptoms such as hallucinations improve. Comprehensive treatment strategies are required to address both symptom categories.

Q129. Answer: A

Explanation: Gradual exposure therapy helps individuals confront feared situations in a controlled and systematic way. The process reduces anxiety by allowing the person to experience the situation without the expected negative outcome. Repeated exposure decreases fear responses over time. This technique is widely used in treating phobias and social anxiety. It promotes confidence and improved coping skills.

Q130. Answer: D

Explanation: Panic disorder involves recurrent, unexpected panic attacks characterized by intense physical and emotional symptoms. Episodes often include shortness of breath, palpitations, dizziness, and overwhelming fear. These attacks may occur without an obvious trigger and can lead to avoidance of certain situations. Persistent concern about future attacks is common. Effective treatment includes psychotherapy and medication when necessary.

Q131. Answer: B

Explanation: Persistent depressive disorder involves long-term depressive symptoms that last for extended periods. Individuals often experience low mood, reduced motivation, and decreased energy. Although symptoms may be less severe than major depression, their chronic nature can significantly impair functioning. Early recognition helps guide appropriate therapeutic interventions. Treatment often combines psychotherapy and medication.

Q132. Answer: C

Explanation: Generalized anxiety disorder is characterized by excessive worry about various aspects of daily life. Physical symptoms frequently accompany the anxiety, including muscle tension, fatigue, and sleep disturbances. Individuals often find it difficult to control the persistent worrying. The condition can interfere with occupational and social functioning. Treatment typically includes therapy, stress management strategies, and medication when necessary.

Q133. Answer: C

Explanation: A delusion of reference occurs when individuals believe unrelated events or communications are directed specifically at them. This belief persists despite clear evidence to the contrary. Such symptoms are commonly seen in psychotic disorders. The experience can cause confusion, distress, and social withdrawal. Proper psychiatric assessment is essential for diagnosis and treatment planning.

Q134. Answer: C

Explanation: Anhedonia refers to the diminished ability to experience pleasure from activities that were previously enjoyable. It is a hallmark symptom of major depressive disorder. Individuals may withdraw from hobbies, relationships, or entertainment they once valued. The loss of interest contributes to decreased motivation and social isolation. Effective treatment focuses on improving mood and restoring engagement in meaningful activities.

Q135. Answer: D

Explanation: Narcissistic personality disorder involves an inflated sense of self-importance and a strong need for admiration. Individuals often believe they possess exceptional abilities or achievements. Interpersonal relationships may be affected due to lack of empathy toward others. These patterns typically begin in early adulthood and persist across many situations. Psychotherapy can help individuals develop healthier interpersonal behaviors.

Q136. Answer: C

Explanation: Dissociative amnesia involves the inability to recall important autobiographical information, often following traumatic or stressful events. The memory loss is not due to neurological damage or substance use. Psychological factors disrupt the normal integration of memory. Individuals may experience confusion about personal history or identity. Treatment focuses on supportive therapy and gradual recovery of memory processes.

Q137. Answer: C

Explanation: Illness anxiety disorder is characterized by persistent fear of having or developing a serious medical condition. Individuals often misinterpret normal bodily sensations as signs of disease. Despite reassurance and normal medical findings, the anxiety continues. The worry can lead to frequent medical visits or excessive health-related behaviors. Psychological treatment helps patients manage these concerns.

Q138. Answer: C

Explanation: Separation anxiety disorder involves excessive fear or distress when separated from attachment figures. Children may worry that harm will come to their caregivers or that they will never reunite. The anxiety can lead to refusal to attend school or participate in activities away from home. Physical complaints such as headaches or stomachaches may accompany the distress. Early intervention helps children develop independence and coping skills.

Q139. Answer: D

Explanation: Antisocial personality disorder is characterized by disregard for social norms and the rights of others. Individuals may engage in deceitful or manipulative behavior for personal gain. Impulsivity and lack of remorse are commonly observed. These patterns often begin in adolescence and continue into adulthood. Treatment focuses on behavioral management and addressing harmful patterns.

Q140. Answer: C

Explanation: Obsessions are intrusive and unwanted thoughts that repeatedly enter a person's mind. They often cause anxiety or distress because they conflict with the individual's values or intentions. People recognize that these thoughts are irrational but feel unable to control them. Obsessions commonly occur in obsessive compulsive disorder. Treatment aims to reduce the frequency and distress associated with these thoughts.

Q141. Answer: B

Explanation: Agoraphobia involves fear of situations where escape may be challenging or help unavailable if anxiety symptoms occur. Individuals frequently avoid crowded locations, public transportation, or open spaces. The avoidance behaviors may significantly limit daily activities. The condition is often associated with panic disorder. Gradual exposure and therapy help individuals regain independence.

Q142. Answer: D

Explanation: Some antidepressants can trigger manic symptoms in individuals with underlying bipolar disorder. Signs may include increased energy, reduced sleep, and impulsive behavior. Early recognition is important to prevent escalation into full mania. Clinicians typically reassess diagnosis and adjust treatment accordingly. Mood stabilizing medications may be required.

Q143. Answer: B

Explanation: Dependent personality disorder involves excessive reliance on others for emotional support and decision-making. Individuals may feel uncomfortable being alone and fear abandonment. They often seek constant reassurance and guidance from caregivers or partners. This dependency can interfere with personal autonomy and healthy relationships. Psychotherapy helps individuals build confidence and independent functioning.

Q144. Answer: D

Explanation: Major depressive disorder involves persistent low mood and loss of interest in activities. Physical symptoms such as fatigue, appetite changes, and sleep disturbances are common. The symptoms must persist for a significant period and interfere with daily functioning. Early recognition allows timely treatment and prevents worsening of the condition. Treatment usually includes psychotherapy, medication, or a combination of both.

Q145. Answer: D

Explanation: Borderline personality disorder often includes emotional instability and difficulty controlling anger. Interpersonal relationships may be intense but unstable. Individuals may react impulsively when feeling rejected or abandoned. These emotional shifts can lead to significant distress and interpersonal conflict. Structured psychotherapy is the primary treatment approach.

Q146. Answer: B

Explanation: Insomnia disorder involves difficulty initiating or maintaining sleep despite adequate opportunity for rest. The condition can lead to daytime fatigue, irritability, and impaired concentration. Chronic sleep disruption may worsen existing mental health conditions. Evaluation typically includes assessment of sleep habits and underlying causes. Treatment may include behavioral therapy and lifestyle modifications.

Q147. Answer: D

Explanation: Panic attacks are sudden surges of intense fear that reach peak intensity within minutes. Physical symptoms often include trembling, sweating, chest discomfort, and dizziness. The experience can be frightening and may occur without warning. Recurrent episodes may lead to development of panic disorder. Treatment focuses on reducing anxiety and preventing future episodes.

Q148. Answer: A

Explanation: Histrionic personality disorder is characterized by excessive emotionality and attention-seeking behavior. Individuals often feel uncomfortable when they are not the center of attention. Their emotional expressions may appear dramatic or exaggerated. Relationships may be shallow because interactions are often driven by the need for approval. Psychotherapy helps individuals develop healthier interpersonal patterns.

Q149. Answer: D

Explanation: Paranoid delusions involve fixed false beliefs that others intend harm or deception. These beliefs persist even when evidence clearly contradicts them. Individuals may misinterpret neutral events as threatening. Such symptoms are commonly associated with psychotic disorders. Proper psychiatric assessment helps determine appropriate treatment.

Q150. Answer: A

Explanation: Depressive disorders involve prolonged low mood and reduced energy levels. Individuals often experience cognitive difficulties such as poor concentration and indecisiveness. Feelings of hopelessness or worthlessness may also occur. These symptoms can interfere with daily functioning and social relationships. Early diagnosis and treatment help improve emotional well-being and restore functioning.

Q151. Answer: A

Explanation: Generalized anxiety disorder involves chronic and excessive worry about various aspects of life. Individuals often feel restless and experience persistent muscle tension and irritability. Concentration difficulties may occur because the mind remains preoccupied with worry. The symptoms typically last for months and interfere with daily functioning. Early recognition allows effective treatment through therapy and medication.

Q152. Answer: C

Explanation: Delirium is an acute disturbance in attention and awareness that develops over a short period. The condition often presents with confusion, disorientation, and fluctuating levels of consciousness. It commonly occurs in medical settings due to infection, medication effects, or metabolic disturbances. Early identification is essential because the underlying cause is often reversible. Prompt treatment helps restore cognitive functioning.

Q153. Answer: C

Explanation: Auditory hallucinations involve hearing sounds or voices without an external stimulus. In schizophrenia, individuals may hear voices conversing or commenting on behavior. These experiences can be highly distressing and may influence behavior or emotional responses. The symptom reflects a disturbance in perception rather than belief. Antipsychotic medications are commonly used to reduce these experiences.

Q154. Answer: C

Explanation: Narcissistic personality disorder involves a persistent pattern of grandiosity and an exaggerated sense of self-importance. Individuals often believe they deserve special treatment and admiration. Empathy toward others may be limited, which can strain relationships. The behavior typically begins in early adulthood and persists across many situations. Psychotherapy focuses on developing healthier interpersonal awareness.

Q155. Answer: D

Explanation: Dissociative amnesia involves the inability to recall important autobiographical information. The memory loss usually occurs after severe psychological stress or trauma. It cannot be explained by neurological injury or substance use. Individuals may become confused about personal history or identity. Therapeutic support helps gradually restore memory integration.

Q156. Answer: D

Explanation: Social anxiety disorder involves a strong fear of negative evaluation by others. Individuals may avoid conversations, meetings, or social gatherings due to fear of embarrassment. Physical symptoms such as sweating and trembling may occur during exposure to social situations. Avoidance behaviors can significantly impair social and occupational functioning. Psychotherapy and medication often help reduce symptoms.

Q157. Answer: B

Explanation: Obsessive compulsive disorder involves intrusive thoughts that produce significant anxiety. Compulsive behaviors are performed to reduce the distress associated with these thoughts. Arranging objects repeatedly is an example of a ritual intended to create a sense of control. These behaviors can become time consuming and interfere with normal activities. Behavioral therapy helps individuals gradually reduce compulsive rituals.

Q158. Answer: D

Explanation: Narcolepsy is a neurological sleep disorder characterized by overwhelming daytime drowsiness. Individuals may suddenly fall asleep during routine activities. These episodes can occur even after adequate nighttime sleep. The condition affects normal regulation of sleep-wake cycles. Medical evaluation and treatment help improve alertness and daily functioning.

Q159. Answer: C

Explanation: Delusions are fixed false beliefs that remain unchanged despite clear contradictory evidence. The belief that a partner is unfaithful without proof is a common example. Such beliefs may lead to conflict and distress in relationships. Delusions typically occur in psychotic disorders or severe mood disorders. Proper psychiatric assessment is required for diagnosis and management.

Q160. Answer: D

Explanation: Somatic symptom disorder involves excessive concern about physical symptoms that lack a clear medical explanation. The distress is real to the patient and often leads to frequent healthcare visits. Individuals may become preoccupied with bodily sensations. The symptoms significantly interfere with daily functioning. Psychological approaches help address the underlying distress and health anxiety.

Q161. Answer: B

Explanation: Schizoid personality disorder involves a pattern of detachment from social relationships. Individuals typically prefer solitary activities and show limited emotional expression. They often appear indifferent to praise or criticism from others. Social interactions may feel uncomfortable or unnecessary to them. Psychotherapy may help improve interpersonal awareness and coping skills.

Q162. Answer: C

Explanation: Post-traumatic stress disorder develops following exposure to a traumatic event. Individuals often experience intrusive recollections and heightened sensitivity to perceived threats. The nervous system remains in a state of hyperarousal, leading to exaggerated startle responses. Avoidance of trauma-related reminders is also common. Early psychological support can reduce long-term psychological impact.

Q163. Answer: D

Explanation: Compulsions are repetitive behaviors performed in response to intrusive thoughts or anxiety. Individuals often recognize that the behavior is excessive but feel compelled to perform it. The act temporarily reduces distress associated with obsessive thoughts. Over time, the ritual can become time-consuming and disruptive. Behavioral therapy helps reduce reliance on these rituals.

Q164. Answer: B

Explanation: Depressive disorders involve persistent emotional distress and mood changes. Individuals may experience unexplained episodes of sadness or tearfulness. These symptoms often occur alongside fatigue, low motivation, and decreased interest in activities. The emotional changes may significantly affect daily functioning. Early treatment improves emotional stability and quality of life.

Q165. Answer: D

Explanation: Avoidant personality disorder involves extreme sensitivity to criticism and fear of rejection. Individuals often desire relationships but avoid them due to fear of embarrassment. Social withdrawal becomes a protective strategy against perceived judgment. The pattern can lead to loneliness and reduced self-confidence. Psychotherapy focuses on building social skills and self-esteem.

Q166. Answer: D

Explanation: Mania is characterized by an elevated or irritable mood accompanied by increased activity and energy. Individuals may speak rapidly and show exaggerated confidence. Sleep requirements decrease without feelings of fatigue. Impulsive behavior may also occur during manic episodes. Mood stabilizing treatment helps control these symptoms.

Q167. Answer: A

Explanation: Major depressive disorder involves prolonged periods of low mood and diminished interest in activities. Individuals may experience fatigue, appetite changes, and difficulty concentrating. Emotional distress can significantly impair social and occupational functioning. The symptoms typically last for weeks or longer. Treatment often includes psychotherapy, medication, or both.

Q168. Answer: C

Explanation: Antisocial personality disorder involves disregard for the rights and feelings of others. Individuals may engage in deceitful or manipulative behaviors for personal benefit. A lack of guilt or remorse often accompanies these actions. The behavior pattern typically begins during adolescence and persists into adulthood. Treatment focuses on behavioral management and improving social responsibility.

Q169. Answer: C

Explanation: Delirium can be triggered by medication effects, especially in vulnerable individuals. The condition involves rapid onset of confusion and changes in attention or awareness. Symptoms often fluctuate throughout the day. Identifying the underlying cause is critical for treatment. Removing the precipitating factor usually leads to improvement.

Q170. Answer: D

Explanation: Histrionic personality disorder is characterized by dramatic emotional expression and strong desire for attention. Individuals may behave in a theatrical or exaggerated manner to gain recognition. Relationships may appear intense but lack depth. Emotional displays may shift quickly depending on the situation. Psychotherapy helps individuals develop more stable interpersonal patterns.

Q171. Answer: B

Explanation: Paranoid delusions involve persistent beliefs that others intend harm or are monitoring the individual. These beliefs continue despite lack of supporting evidence. The perception can lead to mistrust and social withdrawal. Individuals may misinterpret harmless actions as threatening. Professional evaluation is necessary to determine appropriate treatment.

Q172. Answer: A

Explanation: Obsessions are intrusive thoughts or images that repeatedly enter a person's mind. These thoughts are unwanted and cause significant anxiety. Individuals often recognize that the thoughts are irrational but struggle to control them. Obsessions frequently occur in obsessive compulsive disorder. Treatment focuses on reducing the anxiety associated with these thoughts.

Q173. Answer: B

Explanation: Specific phobia involves intense fear of a particular object or situation. Exposure to the feared stimulus often triggers immediate anxiety or panic. Individuals typically avoid the situation whenever possible. The fear is disproportionate to the actual danger posed. Behavioral therapy using gradual exposure is an effective treatment.

Q174. Answer: D

Explanation: Depressive disorders involve emotional and physical symptoms that affect daily functioning. Changes in appetite and sleep are common features. Individuals may feel persistently sad or hopeless for extended periods. These symptoms can interfere with work, relationships, and self-care. Early treatment improves emotional recovery and functioning.

Q175. Answer: C

Explanation: Social anxiety disorder involves a strong fear of embarrassment in social or performance situations. Individuals may avoid public speaking or group discussions. The fear arises from concern about negative evaluation by others. Physical symptoms such as trembling or sweating may accompany the anxiety. Therapy helps individuals gradually confront and manage these fears.

Q176. Answer: B

Explanation: Rapid cycling in bipolar disorder refers to frequent mood episodes within a short period. Individuals may transition quickly between elevated and depressed moods. These fluctuations can significantly disrupt daily functioning. Recognition of the pattern is important for treatment planning. Medication adjustments may be necessary to stabilize mood.

Q177. Answer: D

Explanation: Narcissistic personality disorder includes a persistent pattern of grandiosity and exaggerated self-importance. Individuals may believe they have exceptional talents or achievements. They often seek admiration from others and expect special treatment. Relationships may become strained due to lack of empathy. Psychotherapy focuses on improving self-awareness and interpersonal functioning.

Q178. Answer: B

Explanation: Panic attacks are intense episodes of fear that occur suddenly and peak quickly. Physical symptoms may include heart palpitations, dizziness, and shortness of breath. The experience can be overwhelming and frightening. Recurrent attacks may lead to avoidance behaviors. Treatment focuses on reducing anxiety and preventing future episodes.

Q179. Answer: D

Explanation: Generalized anxiety disorder involves excessive and persistent worry about various aspects of daily life. The worry is difficult to control and occurs most days for extended periods. Individuals may experience restlessness, fatigue, and sleep disturbance. The anxiety can interfere with concentration and productivity. Therapy and medication are commonly used to manage symptoms.

Q180. Answer: B

Explanation: Borderline personality disorder involves instability in emotions, self-image, and relationships. Individuals often fear abandonment and may experience intense emotional reactions. Feelings of emptiness and identity disturbance are common. Interpersonal relationships may shift rapidly between idealization and conflict. Psychotherapy is the primary treatment approach.

Q181. Answer: C

Explanation: Obsessive compulsive disorder includes repetitive behaviors performed to relieve anxiety caused by intrusive thoughts. Counting rituals are common examples of compulsive actions. The behaviors temporarily reduce distress but reinforce the cycle of anxiety. Over time, these rituals may become disruptive to daily activities. Behavioral therapy helps individuals resist and gradually eliminate compulsions.

Q182. Answer: B

Explanation: Somatic symptom disorder involves excessive focus on physical symptoms that cannot be fully explained medically. The distress is genuine and may cause frequent medical visits. Individuals may interpret normal bodily sensations as signs of serious illness. The preoccupation interferes with daily functioning. Psychological treatment addresses health anxiety and coping strategies.

Q183. Answer: C

Explanation: Dissociative amnesia involves memory loss related to traumatic or stressful experiences. The individual cannot recall important autobiographical information. The condition is psychological rather than neurological in origin. Memory gaps may involve specific events or entire periods of life. Therapeutic support helps individuals gradually process and recover memories.

Q184. Answer: C

Explanation: Social anxiety disorder involves fear of being negatively evaluated in social settings. Individuals often avoid conversations or group interactions. The fear can significantly affect occupational and social functioning. Physical symptoms such as trembling or sweating may occur in social situations. Treatment includes psychotherapy and sometimes medication.

Q185. Answer: B

Explanation: Anhedonia refers to the loss of ability to feel pleasure. It is a core symptom of depressive disorders. Activities that were once enjoyable may no longer bring satisfaction. This symptom contributes to withdrawal from hobbies and social interactions. Effective treatment of depression often restores interest in activities.

Q186. Answer: D

Explanation: Paranoid personality disorder involves a pattern of distrust and suspicion of others. Individuals often interpret harmless actions as malicious. Relationships may become strained because the person expects betrayal or exploitation. These beliefs are deeply ingrained and difficult to change. Psychotherapy focuses on improving interpersonal trust and coping strategies.

Q187. Answer: D

Explanation: Borderline personality disorder involves intense emotional instability and difficulty maintaining stable relationships. Individuals may experience rapid mood changes and fear of abandonment. Emotional responses may be disproportionate to the situation. Impulsive behaviors can also occur during periods of distress. Structured psychotherapy helps improve emotional regulation.

Q188. Answer: D

Explanation: Histrionic personality disorder is characterized by attention-seeking behavior and exaggerated emotional expression. Individuals may speak dramatically and behave theatrically in social settings. The desire for attention often influences their interactions with others. Relationships may appear intense but lack emotional depth. Therapy helps individuals develop healthier communication styles.

Q189. Answer: B

Explanation: Dependent personality disorder involves excessive need for reassurance and support from others. Individuals may feel incapable of making decisions independently. Fear of abandonment leads them to seek constant guidance. This reliance can limit personal autonomy and confidence. Psychotherapy helps build independence and self-efficacy.

Q190. Answer: D

Explanation: Obsessions are intrusive and repetitive thoughts that cause significant anxiety. Individuals recognize that these thoughts are unwanted and inconsistent with their values. The distress often leads to attempts to suppress or neutralize the thoughts. Obsessions commonly occur in obsessive compulsive disorder. Treatment focuses on reducing the distress associated with these intrusive thoughts.

Q191. Answer: C

Explanation: Depressive disorders often involve physical symptoms such as fatigue and low energy. Individuals may feel exhausted despite resting adequately. The reduced energy can interfere with work, social interactions, and daily activities. Emotional distress often accompanies these physical symptoms. Treatment addressing mood symptoms usually improves energy levels.

Q192. Answer: A

Explanation: Delirium is an acute change in mental status characterized by confusion and impaired attention. It frequently occurs in hospitalized patients with medical illnesses. The symptoms often fluctuate throughout the day and may worsen at night. Identifying and treating the underlying medical cause is essential. Early management usually leads to improvement.

Q193. Answer: C

Explanation: Delusions are fixed beliefs that remain unchanged despite evidence disproving them. The belief that others are secretly recording conversations reflects paranoid thinking. Such beliefs can cause anxiety and mistrust in relationships. They are commonly associated with psychotic disorders. Psychiatric evaluation is necessary for diagnosis and treatment.

Q194. Answer: A

Explanation: Illness anxiety disorder involves persistent concern about having a serious medical condition. Individuals may repeatedly seek reassurance or medical evaluation. The anxiety continues even when test results show no disease. The worry can significantly affect daily functioning. Psychological interventions help reduce health-related anxiety.

Q195. Answer: C

Explanation: Specific phobias involve intense fear of particular objects or situations. Elevators are a common example of a situational trigger. Exposure to the feared object often produces immediate anxiety. Avoidance behaviors develop to prevent the distressing experience. Behavioral therapy helps individuals gradually overcome the fear.

Q196. Answer: D

Explanation: Cognitive symptoms involve problems with mental processes such as attention, memory, and decision making. Difficulty focusing during conversations reflects impaired concentration. These symptoms may occur in several psychiatric conditions including depression and anxiety. Cognitive impairments can interfere with learning and daily activities. Addressing the underlying disorder often improves cognitive functioning.

Q197. Answer: D

Explanation: Excessive guilt and feelings of worthlessness are common symptoms of depressive disorders. Individuals may interpret minor events as personal failures. These thoughts contribute to low self-esteem and emotional distress. The symptoms often persist for extended periods and interfere with daily functioning. Treatment aims to improve mood and modify negative thinking patterns.

Q198. Answer: A

Explanation: Agoraphobia involves fear of situations where escape might be difficult during anxiety symptoms. Traveling alone or being in unfamiliar places may trigger intense fear. Individuals often avoid these situations to prevent panic experiences. The avoidance can significantly limit independence and mobility. Therapy helps gradually reintroduce feared situations in a controlled way.

Q199. Answer: D

Explanation: Schizoid personality disorder involves detachment from social relationships and limited emotional expression. Individuals typically prefer solitary activities and may appear indifferent to praise or criticism. Emotional responses are often minimal in social interactions. These traits usually begin in early adulthood. Therapy focuses on improving awareness of interpersonal functioning.

Q200. Answer: D

Explanation: Generalized anxiety disorder is characterized by persistent and excessive worry about everyday situations. Physical symptoms such as muscle tension and restlessness commonly accompany the anxiety. Individuals often find it difficult to relax or control the worrying thoughts. The condition typically lasts for months and interferes with daily functioning. Effective treatment includes psychotherapy, stress management techniques, and medication when necessary.

Question (201-300)

Q201. A patient with major depressive disorder reports persistent fatigue, low mood, and diminished concentration for two months. The psychiatric-mental health nurse practitioner recognizes that these symptoms primarily reflect dysfunction in which neurotransmitter system?

(A) Dopamine and norepinephrine pathways
(B) Acetylcholine and glutamate pathways
(C) Histamine and gamma-aminobutyric acid pathways
(D) Serotonin and norepinephrine pathways

Q202. During a psychiatric evaluation, a patient demonstrates rapid shifts in emotional expression and exaggerated theatrical behavior. The nurse practitioner suspects which personality disorder?

(A) Borderline personality disorder
(B) Histrionic personality disorder
(C) Paranoid personality disorder
(D) Narcissistic personality disorder

Q203. A patient receiving lithium therapy reports nausea, mild tremors, and frequent urination. The psychiatric nurse practitioner suspects which condition?

(A) Normal therapeutic effect
(B) Acute renal failure
(C) Lithium withdrawal syndrome
(D) Early lithium toxicity

Q204. A patient experiencing severe anxiety reports heart palpitations, sweating, and trembling during stressful situations. These symptoms are primarily mediated by activation of which system?

(A) Sympathetic nervous system
(B) Enteric nervous system
(C) Parasympathetic nervous system
(D) Somatic nervous system

Q205. A patient states, "I know the government has planted cameras in my house to monitor me." The psychiatric nurse practitioner documents this belief as:

(A) Obsession
(B) Illusion
(C) Delusion
(D) Phobia

Q206. A patient receiving haloperidol develops muscle rigidity, fever, and altered consciousness. The psychiatric nurse practitioner suspects:

(A) Acute dystonic reaction
(B) Neuroleptic malignant syndrome
(C) Serotonin syndrome
(D) Tardive dyskinesia

Q207. During a mental status examination, a patient repeats the last words spoken by the clinician. This phenomenon is called:

(A) Echolalia
(B) Perseveration
(C) Circumstantial speech
(D) Neologism

Q208. A patient with panic disorder asks why symptoms such as dizziness and chest pain occur during panic attacks. The nurse practitioner explains that these symptoms are related to:

(A) Reduced oxygen delivery to the brain

(B) Hyperventilation and autonomic arousal
(C) Excess insulin secretion
(D) Viral infection affecting the nervous system

Q209. A patient reports persistent intrusive thoughts about contamination and spends hours washing their hands each day. The psychiatric nurse practitioner recognizes these symptoms as:

(A) Illness anxiety disorder
(B) Generalized anxiety disorder
(C) Obsessive-compulsive disorder
(D) Body dysmorphic disorder

Q210. A patient treated with selective serotonin reuptake inhibitors develops agitation, sweating, confusion, and muscle twitching. The psychiatric nurse practitioner suspects:

(A) Acute dystonia
(B) Serotonin syndrome
(C) Lithium toxicity
(D) Neuroleptic malignant syndrome

Q211. A patient demonstrates decreased need for sleep, inflated self-esteem, and excessive involvement in risky activities. These symptoms suggest:

(A) Major depressive episode
(B) Cyclothymic disorder
(C) Manic episode
(D) Hypomanic episode

Q212. A patient with schizophrenia reports hearing voices that comment on their behavior throughout the day. This symptom represents:

(A) Thought insertion
(B) Auditory hallucination
(C) Visual hallucination
(D) Somatic delusion

Q213. A patient taking clozapine requires regular blood monitoring primarily due to the risk of:

(A) Hypertension
(B) Hypokalemia
(C) Agranulocytosis
(D) Hyperglycemia

Q214. A patient reports persistent sadness following the death of a spouse two months ago but continues normal daily activities. The psychiatric nurse practitioner recognizes this as:

(A) Major depressive disorder
(B) Normal grief response
(C) Adjustment disorder with psychosis
(D) Persistent depressive disorder

Q215. A patient with alcohol use disorder presents with tremors, sweating, and agitation twelve hours after the last drink. These symptoms indicate:

(A) Alcohol withdrawal
(B) Hepatic encephalopathy
(C) Alcohol intoxication
(D) Alcohol-induced psychosis

Q216. During therapy, a patient attributes their own unacceptable feelings to another person. This defense mechanism is known as:

(A) Reaction formation
(B) Sublimation

(C) Projection
(D) Displacement

Q217. A patient taking benzodiazepines for several months suddenly stops the medication and develops anxiety, insomnia, and tremors. The nurse practitioner recognizes this as:
(A) Medication tolerance
(B) Drug allergy
(C) Withdrawal syndrome
(D) Placebo effect

Q218. A patient experiencing major depression begins treatment with an antidepressant medication. The nurse practitioner explains that noticeable symptom improvement typically occurs after:
(A) 48 hours
(B) 24 hours
(C) 6 hours
(D) 2-4 weeks

Q219. During a psychiatric interview, a patient answers questions with excessive unnecessary detail but eventually returns to the main point. This speech pattern is described as:
(A) Flight of ideas
(B) Circumstantial speech
(C) Tangential speech
(D) Word salad

Q220. A patient undergoing cognitive behavioral therapy learns to identify and challenge negative automatic thoughts. The primary goal of this therapy is to:
(A) Increase medication adherence
(B) Explore childhood trauma
(C) Modify unconscious conflicts
(D) Change maladaptive thought patterns

Q221. A patient experiencing persistent anxiety reports muscle tension, restlessness, and difficulty concentrating for more than six months. These symptoms most strongly suggest:
(A) Panic disorder
(B) Acute stress disorder
(C) Social anxiety disorder
(D) Generalized anxiety disorder

Q222. A patient reports repeated episodes of binge eating followed by self-induced vomiting to prevent weight gain. The psychiatric nurse practitioner recognizes this condition as:
(A) Anorexia nervosa
(B) Binge eating disorder
(C) Avoidant restrictive food intake disorder
(D) Bulimia nervosa

Q223. A patient taking antipsychotic medication develops sustained muscle contractions of the neck and face shortly after starting therapy. The psychiatric nurse practitioner identifies this as:
(A) Tardive dyskinesia
(B) Akathisia
(C) Acute dystonia
(D) Neuroleptic malignant syndrome

Q224. A patient reports persistent fear of being judged or embarrassed when speaking in public or meeting unfamiliar people. This presentation is most consistent with:
(A) Specific phobia
(B) Agoraphobia

(C) Panic disorder
(D) Social anxiety disorder

Q225. A patient reports episodes of intense fear accompanied by chest pain, shortness of breath, and feelings of impending doom that reach a peak within minutes. These symptoms indicate:
(A) Dissociative episode
(B) Adjustment reaction
(C) Generalized anxiety episode
(D) Panic attack

Q226. A patient with schizophrenia demonstrates minimal facial expression, reduced speech, and lack of motivation. These symptoms are categorized as:
(A) Cognitive symptoms
(B) Positive symptoms
(C) Affective symptoms
(D) Negative symptoms

Q227. A patient with bipolar disorder is prescribed valproate. The psychiatric nurse practitioner monitors which laboratory parameter most closely?
(A) Thyroid function
(B) Serum calcium
(C) Liver function tests
(D) Blood glucose

Q228. A patient with post-traumatic stress disorder reports recurrent nightmares and intrusive memories related to a traumatic event. These symptoms represent:
(A) Hyperarousal symptoms
(B) Intrusion symptoms
(C) Dissociative symptoms
(D) Avoidance symptoms

Q229. A patient persistently checks door locks and appliances repeatedly due to fear that something terrible will occur if they do not. The behavior is best described as:
(A) Delusion
(B) Obsession
(C) Impulse
(D) Compulsion

Q230. A patient reports a persistent depressed mood lasting more than two years with only brief periods of symptom relief. This presentation is most consistent with:
(A) Adjustment disorder
(B) Major depressive disorder
(C) Persistent depressive disorder
(D) Cyclothymic disorder

Q231. A patient believes their thoughts are being controlled by an external force. This symptom represents:
(A) Thought broadcasting
(B) Grandiose delusion
(C) Thought insertion
(D) Delusion of control

Q232. A patient experiencing alcohol withdrawal develops confusion, agitation, and vivid visual hallucinations. These symptoms indicate:
(A) Wernicke encephalopathy
(B) Korsakoff syndrome

(C) Alcohol intoxication
(D) Delirium tremens

Q233. A patient consistently exaggerates physical symptoms despite normal medical evaluations. The psychiatric nurse practitioner considers:
(A) Illness anxiety disorder
(B) Somatic symptom disorder
(C) Factitious disorder
(D) Conversion disorder

Q234. A patient demonstrates persistent irritability and frequent temper outbursts occurring several times per week for over a year. The nurse practitioner considers:
(A) Disruptive mood dysregulation disorder
(B) Oppositional defiant disorder
(C) Conduct disorder
(D) Attention deficit hyperactivity disorder

Q235. A patient repeatedly pulls out their hair resulting in noticeable hair loss. This condition is known as:
(A) Excoriation disorder
(B) Body dysmorphic disorder
(C) Trichotillomania
(D) Dermatillomania

Q236. A patient experiences sudden episodes of intense anger and aggression that are disproportionate to the situation. The nurse practitioner suspects:
(A) Antisocial personality disorder
(B) Conduct disorder
(C) Intermittent explosive disorder
(D) Oppositional defiant disorder

Q237. A patient experiences recurrent episodes of sleep paralysis when falling asleep or waking. This condition is associated with:
(A) Sleep apnea
(B) Insomnia disorder
(C) Restless leg syndrome
(D) Narcolepsy

Q238. A patient persistently lies, manipulates others, and shows little remorse for harmful actions. These behaviors suggest:
(A) Narcissistic personality disorder
(B) Antisocial personality disorder
(C) Borderline personality disorder
(D) Dependent personality disorder

Q239. A patient complains of persistent difficulty falling asleep despite adequate opportunity to sleep. This condition is most consistent with:
(A) Circadian rhythm disorder
(B) Parasomnia
(C) Insomnia disorder
(D) Hypersomnia disorder

Q240. A patient becomes extremely anxious when separated from close family members and fears harm will occur to them. This presentation suggests:
(A) Specific phobia
(B) Separation anxiety disorder

(C) Social anxiety disorder
(D) Panic disorder

Q241. A patient frequently complains of multiple physical symptoms including headaches, stomach pain, and fatigue that cannot be fully explained by medical evaluation. The psychiatric nurse practitioner considers:
(A) Factitious disorder
(B) Somatic symptom disorder
(C) Illness anxiety disorder
(D) Conversion disorder

Q242. A patient reports experiencing a sudden inability to move their arm after witnessing a traumatic event, but neurological testing shows no physical cause. This condition is best described as:
(A) Conversion disorder
(B) Somatic symptom disorder
(C) Factitious disorder
(D) Illness anxiety disorder

Q243. A patient repeatedly seeks medical treatment and intentionally falsifies symptoms in order to assume the sick role. This presentation suggests:
(A) Somatic symptom disorder
(B) Factitious disorder
(C) Malingering
(D) Illness anxiety disorder

Q244. A patient persistently believes they have a serious illness despite repeated medical reassurance and minimal symptoms. The psychiatric nurse practitioner suspects:
(A) Illness anxiety disorder
(B) Conversion disorder
(C) Delusional disorder
(D) Somatic symptom disorder

Q245. A patient experiencing hallucinations and disorganized speech for one month following a severe stressor most likely meets criteria for:
(A) Schizophrenia
(B) Brief psychotic disorder
(C) Delusional disorder
(D) Schizoaffective disorder

Q246. A patient demonstrates symptoms of psychosis for eight months including hallucinations, disorganized behavior, and social withdrawal. The most likely diagnosis is:
(A) Delusional disorder
(B) Brief psychotic disorder
(C) Schizophreniform disorder
(D) Schizophrenia

Q247. A patient reports persistent depressed mood accompanied by episodes of elevated mood that do not meet criteria for mania or major depression. The nurse practitioner suspects:
(A) Bipolar II disorder
(B) Cyclothymic disorder
(C) Persistent depressive disorder
(D) Bipolar I disorder

Q248. A patient with bipolar disorder experiences episodes of major depression alternating with hypomania but has never experienced full mania. The diagnosis is:
(A) Cyclothymic disorder

(B) Persistent depressive disorder
(C) Bipolar I disorder
(D) Bipolar II disorder

Q249. A patient experiences recurrent thoughts about harming a loved one despite having no desire to act on these thoughts. The psychiatric nurse practitioner identifies these thoughts as:
(A) Intrusive thoughts
(B) Hallucinations
(C) Delusions
(D) Phobias

Q250. A patient suddenly becomes extremely anxious when entering elevators and avoids them whenever possible. This behavior most likely represents:
(A) Specific phobia
(B) Panic disorder
(C) Social anxiety disorder
(D) Agoraphobia

Q251. A patient experiences intense fear of leaving home because escape might be difficult if panic symptoms occur. The psychiatric nurse practitioner suspects:
(A) Social anxiety disorder
(B) Generalized anxiety disorder
(C) Specific phobia
(D) Agoraphobia

Q252. A patient reports sudden episodes of uncontrollable eating followed by feelings of shame but does not engage in purging behaviors. This condition is known as:
(A) Bulimia nervosa
(B) Binge eating disorder
(C) Anorexia nervosa
(D) Avoidant restrictive food intake disorder

Q253. A patient with anorexia nervosa demonstrates an intense fear of gaining weight despite being significantly underweight. This symptom represents:
(A) Delusional perception
(B) Cognitive impairment
(C) Body dysmorphic belief
(D) Distorted body image

Q254. A patient repeatedly picks at skin lesions resulting in tissue damage. This behavior is most consistent with:
(A) Conversion disorder
(B) Excoriation disorder
(C) Body dysmorphic disorder
(D) Trichotillomania

Q255. A patient demonstrates a long-standing pattern of excessive need to be taken care of and difficulty making decisions without reassurance. The nurse practitioner suspects:
(A) Avoidant personality disorder
(B) Dependent personality disorder
(C) Borderline personality disorder
(D) Narcissistic personality disorder

Q256. A patient consistently avoids social interactions due to feelings of inadequacy and fear of criticism. This presentation suggests:
(A) Avoidant personality disorder

(B) Paranoid personality disorder
(C) Schizoid personality disorder
(D) Dependent personality disorder

Q257. A patient shows little interest in relationships and prefers solitary activities. Emotional expression appears limited. The nurse practitioner considers:

(A) Schizotypal personality disorder
(B) Schizoid personality disorder
(C) Paranoid personality disorder
(D) Narcissistic personality disorder

Q258. A patient exhibits eccentric behavior, unusual beliefs, and discomfort with close relationships. The psychiatric nurse practitioner suspects:

(A) Schizotypal personality disorder
(B) Schizoid personality disorder
(C) Paranoid personality disorder
(D) Avoidant personality disorder

Q259. A patient persistently suspects that others intend to harm or deceive them without sufficient evidence. This pattern suggests:

(A) Antisocial personality disorder
(B) Narcissistic personality disorder
(C) Borderline personality disorder
(D) Paranoid personality disorder

Q260. A patient displays unstable relationships, impulsivity, and intense fear of abandonment. The psychiatric nurse practitioner recognizes this pattern as:

(A) Borderline personality disorder
(B) Narcissistic personality disorder
(C) Dependent personality disorder
(D) Histrionic personality disorder

Q261. A patient with schizophrenia displays disorganized speech characterized by rapidly shifting topics with only loose associations between ideas. This pattern is known as:

(A) Tangentiality
(B) Circumstantial speech
(C) Flight of ideas
(D) Loose associations

Q262. A patient taking an antipsychotic medication complains of an intense inner restlessness and inability to remain still. The psychiatric nurse practitioner recognizes this condition as:

(A) Dystonia
(B) Parkinsonism
(C) Tardive dyskinesia
(D) Akathisia

Q263. A patient suddenly develops repetitive, involuntary facial movements and lip smacking after long-term use of antipsychotic medication. This presentation suggests:

(A) Akathisia
(B) Parkinsonism
(C) Acute dystonia
(D) Tardive dyskinesia

Q264. A patient reports hearing voices that instruct them to perform certain actions. These experiences are classified as:

(A) Visual hallucinations

(B) Delusional perceptions
(C) Illusions
(D) Command hallucinations

Q265. A patient suddenly stops speaking in the middle of a sentence and is unable to recall what they were saying. This thought disturbance is called:
(A) Neologism
(B) Thought blocking
(C) Circumstantial thinking
(D) Tangential speech

Q266. A patient invents new words that have meaning only to them during conversation. This speech pattern is known as:
(A) Perseveration
(B) Neologism
(C) Clang association
(D) Echolalia

Q267. A patient repeatedly returns to the same word or phrase during conversation despite attempts to move to new topics. This phenomenon is called:
(A) Echolalia
(B) Perseveration
(C) Flight of ideas
(D) Circumstantiality

Q268. A patient experiences episodes of intense fear triggered by encountering spiders. The nurse practitioner identifies this as:
(A) Specific phobia
(B) Panic disorder
(C) Agoraphobia
(D) Social anxiety disorder

Q269. A patient frequently experiences sudden episodes of binge eating late at night without awareness and later finds evidence of food consumption. This condition is known as:
(A) Sleep-related eating disorder
(B) Binge eating disorder
(C) Night eating syndrome
(D) Bulimia nervosa

Q270. A patient repeatedly expresses exaggerated emotional displays and uses dramatic language to describe minor events. The psychiatric nurse practitioner considers:
(A) Narcissistic personality disorder
(B) Borderline personality disorder
(C) Histrionic personality disorder
(D) Dependent personality disorder

Q271. A patient demonstrates an inflated sense of self-importance and expects constant admiration from others. The nurse practitioner suspects:
(A) Narcissistic personality disorder
(B) Avoidant personality disorder
(C) Borderline personality disorder
(D) Dependent personality disorder

Q272. A patient shows a pervasive pattern of emotional instability, impulsivity, and intense interpersonal conflicts. This presentation suggests:
(A) Antisocial personality disorder

(B) Schizoid personality disorder
(C) Borderline personality disorder
(D) Dependent personality disorder

Q273. A patient demonstrates repetitive hand washing and persistent thoughts about contamination. These behaviors indicate:
(A) Illness anxiety disorder
(B) Panic disorder
(C) Obsessive-compulsive disorder
(D) Generalized anxiety disorder

Q274. A patient reports persistent difficulty concentrating, irritability, and hypervigilance after surviving a serious accident. These symptoms are most consistent with:
(A) Post-traumatic stress disorder
(B) Adjustment disorder
(C) Panic disorder
(D) Acute stress disorder

Q275. A patient experiences persistent sadness and loss of interest in activities previously enjoyed for over two weeks. This presentation indicates:
(A) Bipolar disorder
(B) Adjustment disorder
(C) Cyclothymic disorder
(D) Major depressive disorder

Q276. A patient with bipolar disorder demonstrates excessive energy, decreased need for sleep, and rapid speech lasting one week. The nurse practitioner identifies this episode as:
(A) Mania
(B) Hypomania
(C) Cyclothymia
(D) Major depression

Q277. A patient complains of persistent fatigue, weight gain, and depressed mood. Laboratory testing reveals low thyroid hormone levels. The psychiatric nurse practitioner recognizes:
(A) Bipolar disorder
(B) Cyclothymic disorder
(C) Mood disorder due to medical condition
(D) Substance-induced depression

Q278. A patient complains of persistent fear that their body emits an unpleasant odor despite reassurance from others. The nurse practitioner suspects:
(A) Somatic symptom disorder
(B) Delusional disorder
(C) Body dysmorphic disorder
(D) Obsessive-compulsive disorder

Q279. A patient demonstrates persistent difficulty paying attention, excessive activity, and impulsive behavior beginning in childhood. The psychiatric nurse practitioner considers:
(A) Conduct disorder
(B) Disruptive mood dysregulation disorder
(C) Oppositional defiant disorder
(D) Attention-deficit hyperactivity disorder

Q280. A patient repeatedly violates the rights of others and engages in unlawful behavior without remorse. This pattern suggests:
(A) Antisocial personality disorder

(B) Narcissistic personality disorder
(C) Paranoid personality disorder
(D) Borderline personality disorder

Q281. A patient reports episodes of sleepwalking during which they leave the bed and perform activities while still asleep. This condition is classified as:
(A) Circadian rhythm disorder
(B) Insomnia disorder
(C) Parasomnia
(D) Hypersomnia disorder

Q282. A patient persistently worries about everyday issues such as finances, work performance, and family responsibilities. These symptoms are characteristic of:
(A) Panic disorder
(B) Social anxiety disorder
(C) Specific phobia
(D) Generalized anxiety disorder

Q283. A patient begins experiencing hallucinations and delusions shortly after heavy substance use. The psychiatric nurse practitioner considers:
(A) Schizophrenia
(B) Brief psychotic disorder
(C) Substance-induced psychotic disorder
(D) Delusional disorder

Q284. A patient reports experiencing vivid hallucinations just before falling asleep. These are referred to as:
(A) Visual illusions
(B) Hypnagogic hallucinations
(C) Delusional perceptions
(D) Hypnopompic hallucinations

Q285. A patient experiences hallucinations that occur when waking from sleep. These are called:
(A) Hypnopompic hallucinations
(B) Somatic hallucinations
(C) Visual illusions
(D) Hypnagogic hallucinations

Q286. A patient states that the television news anchors are sending them secret messages. This belief is best described as:
(A) Delusion of reference
(B) Delusion of grandeur
(C) Somatic delusion
(D) Nihilistic delusion

Q287. A patient believes they possess extraordinary abilities and immense power beyond ordinary human capability. This symptom represents:
(A) Somatic delusion
(B) Grandiose delusion
(C) Nihilistic delusion
(D) Delusion of persecution

Q288. A patient strongly believes that others are plotting to harm them without evidence. This belief is categorized as:
(A) Somatic delusion
(B) Nihilistic delusion

(C) Delusion of reference
(D) Delusion of persecution
Q289. A patient believes that their organs have stopped functioning despite medical evidence to the contrary. This belief is known as:
(A) Somatic delusion
(B) Nihilistic delusion
(C) Grandiose delusion
(D) Referential delusion
Q290. A patient becomes extremely anxious when exposed to heights and avoids high places whenever possible. The nurse practitioner identifies this as:
(A) Social anxiety disorder
(B) Panic disorder
(C) Specific phobia
(D) Agoraphobia
Q291. A patient reports hearing music when no external sound is present. This experience is classified as:
(A) Delusional perception
(B) Somatic hallucination
(C) Illusion
(D) Auditory hallucination
Q292. A patient misinterprets the shadow of a coat hanging in a dark room as a threatening figure. This perceptual disturbance is known as:
(A) Derealization
(B) Delusion
(C) Illusion
(D) Hallucination
Q293. A patient reports feeling detached from their surroundings as if the world is unreal. This experience is known as:
(A) Dissociation
(B) Hallucination
(C) Depersonalization
(D) Derealization
Q294. A patient describes feeling detached from their own body and emotions as if observing themselves from outside. This phenomenon is called:
(A) Dissociation
(B) Derealization
(C) Depersonalization
(D) Somatization
Q295. A patient repeatedly refuses to speak despite having the ability to do so. This behavior is known as:
(A) Neologism
(B) Catatonia
(C) Mutism
(D) Echolalia
Q296. A patient maintains a rigid posture for long periods and resists attempts to reposition their body. This symptom suggests:
(A) Catatonia
(B) Akathisia

(C) Dystonia
(D) Tardive dyskinesia

Q297. A patient suddenly begins speaking rapidly with ideas changing quickly from one topic to another. This speech pattern is called:
(A) Flight of ideas
(B) Circumstantial speech
(C) Thought blocking
(D) Tangential speech

Q298. A patient answers questions with irrelevant responses and never returns to the original topic. This speech disturbance is known as:
(A) Neologism
(B) Tangential speech
(C) Perseveration
(D) Circumstantial speech

Q299. A patient describes experiencing an exaggerated sense of personal importance and entitlement to special treatment. This characteristic is most associated with:
(A) Schizoid personality disorder
(B) Dependent personality disorder
(C) Narcissistic personality disorder
(D) Avoidant personality disorder

Q300. A patient suddenly develops confusion, fluctuating consciousness, and disorganized thinking after a severe infection. The psychiatric nurse practitioner identifies this condition as:
(A) Bipolar disorder
(B) Dementia
(C) Delirium
(D) Schizophrenia

Answer Key and Explanation (201-300)

Q201. Answer: D

Explanation: Major depressive disorder is strongly associated with dysregulation of serotonin and norepinephrine neurotransmission in the brain. These neurotransmitters influence mood regulation, sleep patterns, appetite, and cognitive processing. Reduced serotonergic activity is linked to sadness and emotional instability, while reduced norepinephrine affects energy and alertness. Antidepressant medications often work by increasing the availability of these neurotransmitters in the synaptic cleft. Improvement in mood symptoms commonly occurs once neurotransmitter balance is partially restored. Neurobiological research consistently supports the involvement of these pathways in depressive disorders.

Q202. Answer: B

Explanation: Histrionic personality disorder is characterized by excessive emotionality and attention-seeking behavior. Individuals frequently display dramatic, theatrical, and exaggerated expressions of emotion. They often feel uncomfortable when they are not the center of attention and may behave in ways designed to attract notice. Interpersonal interactions may appear shallow or rapidly shifting in emotional tone. The behavior pattern usually begins by early adulthood and occurs across various social contexts. Recognition of these traits is essential for accurate diagnosis and therapeutic planning.

Q203. Answer: D

Explanation: Lithium toxicity can occur even within therapeutic ranges if patient physiology changes or drug interactions occur. Early symptoms commonly include gastrointestinal upset, tremor, and increased thirst or urination. These symptoms develop because lithium affects electrolyte balance and neuronal signaling. Monitoring serum lithium levels and renal function is essential to prevent progression to severe toxicity. Without intervention, neurological symptoms such as confusion and ataxia may develop. Prompt recognition helps prevent serious complications.

Q204. Answer: A

Explanation: Anxiety triggers activation of the sympathetic branch of the autonomic nervous system. This system prepares the body for a fight-or-flight response during perceived threats. Physiological effects include increased heart rate, elevated blood pressure, sweating, and heightened alertness. Stress hormones such as epinephrine and norepinephrine are released during this response. These changes enhance the body's ability to react quickly to danger. Persistent activation can contribute to chronic anxiety disorders.

Q205. Answer: C

Explanation: A delusion is a fixed false belief that persists despite clear contradictory evidence. It is typically not shared by members of the patient's cultural or social group. Delusions often occur in psychotic disorders and involve themes such as persecution, grandiosity, or control. The belief remains strongly held even when logical explanations are presented. Assessment should include evaluating the impact on functioning and safety. Treatment usually involves antipsychotic medications and supportive therapy.

Q206. Answer: B

Explanation: Neuroleptic malignant syndrome is a rare but life-threatening reaction associated with antipsychotic medications. It is characterized by hyperthermia, muscle rigidity, autonomic instability, and altered mental status. The condition results from dopamine blockade in the central nervous system. Early recognition is critical because it can rapidly progress to severe complications. Immediate discontinuation of the offending medication and supportive medical treatment are required. Medications such as dantrolene or bromocriptine may be used in severe cases.

Q207. Answer: A

Explanation: Echolalia refers to the automatic repetition of words or phrases spoken by another person. It is often observed in certain psychiatric or neurodevelopmental disorders. This behavior may occur in conditions such as autism spectrum disorder or schizophrenia. It represents an abnormality in language processing and communication. Assessment should consider the broader context of speech patterns and cognitive functioning. Understanding the behavior helps guide appropriate therapeutic interventions.

Q208. Answer: B

Explanation: Panic attacks involve sudden activation of the body's stress response system. Rapid breathing during hyperventilation decreases carbon dioxide levels in the blood. This physiological change can cause dizziness, tingling, and feelings of unreality. Autonomic arousal also leads to increased heart rate and chest discomfort. These symptoms are frightening but generally not medically dangerous. Education about the physiological basis helps reduce fear and improve coping strategies.

Q209. Answer: C

Explanation: Obsessive-compulsive disorder involves intrusive thoughts known as obsessions and repetitive behaviors called compulsions. Obsessions create intense anxiety and distress. Compulsions are performed to reduce anxiety or prevent feared outcomes. The behaviors often become time-consuming and interfere with daily functioning. Neurobiological research links the disorder to dysfunction in cortico-striatal circuits. Treatment typically involves cognitive behavioral therapy and medications that increase serotonin availability.

Q210. Answer: B

Explanation: Serotonin syndrome occurs when excessive serotonergic activity develops in the central nervous system. It is often triggered by medication interactions or high doses of serotonergic drugs. Symptoms include agitation, hyperreflexia, sweating, tremor, and altered mental status. The condition can escalate rapidly if untreated. Immediate discontinuation of serotonergic medications and supportive care are essential. Early intervention usually leads to rapid symptom resolution.

Q211. Answer: C

Explanation: A manic episode involves a period of abnormally elevated or irritable mood accompanied by increased energy and activity. Individuals may sleep very little without feeling fatigued. Grandiosity, impulsive decision-making, and risk-taking behaviors are common. The episode typically causes significant impairment in social or occupational functioning. Hospitalization may be required if safety becomes a concern. Mood stabilizing medications are often necessary to manage symptoms.

Q212. Answer: B

Explanation: Auditory hallucinations involve perceiving sounds or voices without an external stimulus. They are among the most common psychotic symptoms in schizophrenia. The voices may comment on actions, issue commands, or engage in conversation. These experiences feel very real to the individual experiencing them. Neuroimaging studies suggest abnormal activation in auditory processing areas of the brain. Treatment typically includes antipsychotic medications and psychosocial support.

Q213. Answer: C

Explanation: Clozapine is associated with a rare but serious adverse effect involving severe reduction of white blood cells. This condition significantly increases the risk of infection. Because of this risk, routine blood monitoring is required during treatment. Early detection allows prompt discontinuation before severe complications develop. Despite the risk, clozapine is highly effective for treatment-resistant schizophrenia. Careful monitoring allows safe use of the medication in appropriate patients.

Q214. Answer: B

Explanation: Grief following the loss of a loved one is a natural emotional response. Individuals may experience sadness, longing, and occasional sleep disturbance during the grieving process. However, many continue to maintain daily responsibilities and social connections. The emotional experience typically fluctuates and gradually improves with time. Clinical assessment focuses on identifying signs of complicated grief or major depression. Supportive counseling may help individuals process their loss.

Q215. Answer: A

Explanation: Alcohol withdrawal occurs when a person who has been consuming alcohol heavily suddenly stops drinking. The nervous system becomes hyperactive due to loss of the depressant effects of alcohol. Early symptoms include tremor, anxiety, sweating, and agitation. If untreated, withdrawal may progress to seizures or delirium tremens. Early recognition allows timely administration of medications to prevent severe complications. Medical monitoring is often required during the withdrawal process.

Q216. Answer: C

Explanation: Projection is a psychological defense mechanism in which individuals attribute their own unacceptable thoughts or feelings to others. This process allows the person to avoid recognizing these feelings within themselves. It often occurs unconsciously and may distort perception of interpersonal interactions. Projection is frequently observed in certain personality disorders and psychotic conditions. Understanding defense mechanisms can help clinicians interpret behavior patterns during therapy. Awareness also assists in guiding psychotherapeutic interventions.

Q217. Answer: C

Explanation: Long-term benzodiazepine use can lead to physical dependence. Abrupt discontinuation may cause withdrawal symptoms due to neurochemical adaptations in the brain. These symptoms often include anxiety, insomnia, tremors, and irritability. In severe cases, seizures may occur. Gradual tapering of the medication is recommended to reduce withdrawal risk. Monitoring during discontinuation helps ensure patient safety.

Q218. Answer: D

Explanation: Antidepressant medications generally require several weeks before significant clinical improvement becomes noticeable. Although neurotransmitter changes occur rapidly after administration, downstream neuroadaptive processes take longer. These changes involve receptor regulation and altered neural connectivity. Patients should be educated about the delayed onset to prevent premature discontinuation. Adherence during the early phase of treatment is critical for therapeutic success. Regular follow-up helps evaluate effectiveness and adjust treatment when necessary.

Q219. Answer: B

Explanation: Circumstantial speech involves providing excessive and unnecessary detail before eventually arriving at the intended point. The main topic is not completely lost, but the path to the answer is indirect. This pattern may be observed in various psychiatric conditions. It reflects disturbances in thought organization rather than complete derailment. Clinical assessment considers context, severity, and associated symptoms. Understanding speech patterns contributes to accurate mental status evaluation.

Q220. Answer: D

Explanation: Cognitive behavioral therapy focuses on identifying distorted or maladaptive patterns of thinking. These thoughts influence emotions and behaviors in daily life. By learning to challenge and restructure these patterns, patients can reduce psychological distress. The therapy is structured, goal-oriented, and supported by strong research evidence. Many mood and anxiety disorders respond well to this approach. Skills learned during therapy help individuals manage future stressors effectively.

Q221. Answer: D

Explanation: Generalized anxiety disorder involves chronic and excessive worry occurring most days for at least six months. Individuals experience difficulty controlling their anxiety across multiple life areas. Physical symptoms frequently include muscle tension, fatigue, restlessness, and sleep disturbance. Cognitive symptoms such as difficulty concentrating are also common. The disorder significantly interferes with daily functioning and quality of life. Treatment usually includes psychotherapy, lifestyle interventions, and pharmacologic therapy.

Q222. Answer: D

Explanation: Bulimia nervosa is characterized by recurrent episodes of binge eating accompanied by compensatory behaviors aimed at preventing weight gain. These behaviors often include vomiting, misuse of laxatives, excessive exercise, or fasting. Individuals typically maintain body weight within or near the normal range. Feelings of shame and lack of control frequently accompany binge episodes. The disorder can lead to electrolyte imbalances and gastrointestinal complications. Early treatment helps prevent long-term medical and psychological consequences.

Q223. Answer: C

Explanation: Acute dystonia is a movement disorder involving sudden, sustained muscle contractions. These reactions commonly affect muscles of the face, neck, or back. They often occur shortly after initiating or increasing antipsychotic medications. The underlying mechanism involves dopamine blockade within the basal ganglia. Symptoms may be distressing but are typically reversible with prompt treatment. Anticholinergic medications are commonly used to relieve the muscle spasms.

Q224. Answer: D

Explanation: Social anxiety disorder involves intense fear of social situations in which the individual may be evaluated by others. The fear often centers on embarrassment, humiliation, or negative judgment. Situations such as public speaking or meeting new people frequently trigger anxiety. Individuals may avoid social interactions to reduce distress. This avoidance can significantly interfere with occupational and interpersonal functioning. Treatment often includes cognitive behavioral therapy and pharmacologic management.

Q225. Answer: D

Explanation: Panic attacks involve sudden surges of intense fear or discomfort that peak within minutes. Symptoms frequently include chest pain, palpitations, shortness of breath, dizziness, and fear of losing control. The experience may occur unexpectedly or in response to specific triggers. Although frightening, panic attacks are not usually life-threatening. Recurrent episodes can lead to panic disorder when persistent concern about future attacks develops. Early recognition helps guide effective treatment strategies.

Q226. Answer: D

Explanation: Negative symptoms involve reductions or losses in normal emotional and behavioral functioning. Examples include diminished emotional expression, decreased speech output, and reduced motivation. These symptoms can significantly impair social and occupational functioning. They differ from positive symptoms, which involve excesses such as hallucinations or delusions. Negative symptoms are often more difficult to treat and may persist despite medication. Comprehensive management may require psychosocial rehabilitation and supportive therapy.

Q227. Answer: C

Explanation: Valproate is widely used as a mood stabilizer for bipolar disorder. One of the important potential adverse effects involves liver toxicity. Monitoring liver function helps detect early signs of hepatic impairment. Periodic blood tests are recommended during treatment. Early identification of abnormalities allows prompt adjustment or discontinuation of therapy. Safe medication management requires consistent laboratory monitoring.

Q228. Answer: B

Explanation: Intrusion symptoms involve the involuntary re-experiencing of traumatic events. These experiences may occur through distressing memories, flashbacks, or nightmares. The symptoms are often triggered by reminders associated with the trauma. Individuals may feel as though the event is happening again. These experiences can cause significant emotional distress and physiological arousal. Treatment often includes trauma-focused psychotherapy and appropriate medications.

Q229. Answer: D

Explanation: Compulsions are repetitive behaviors performed in response to intrusive thoughts or anxiety. Individuals engage in these actions to reduce distress or prevent feared outcomes. Although the person may recognize the behavior as excessive, they often feel unable to resist performing it. The behaviors can become time-consuming and interfere with daily activities. Compulsions are a core feature of obsessive-compulsive disorder. Effective treatment frequently combines psychotherapy with medication.

Q230. Answer: C

Explanation: Persistent depressive disorder involves chronic depressive symptoms lasting at least two years in adults. The mood disturbance is less severe than major depressive episodes but more prolonged. Individuals often describe feeling consistently down or lacking energy. The chronic nature of symptoms can significantly affect self-esteem and daily functioning. Many individuals also experience episodes of more severe depression during the course of the disorder. Long-term treatment strategies are often necessary.

Q231. Answer: D

Explanation: A delusion of control involves the belief that external forces are controlling one's thoughts, actions, or feelings. This belief is firmly held despite lack of evidence. Such experiences are commonly associated with psychotic disorders. The perception of lost personal autonomy can be very distressing. Clinicians assess the severity and impact of these beliefs on functioning. Antipsychotic medications often help reduce these symptoms.

Q232. Answer: D

Explanation: Delirium tremens is a severe complication of alcohol withdrawal. It typically occurs several days after cessation of heavy alcohol use. Symptoms include confusion, agitation, hallucinations, and autonomic instability. Without treatment, the condition can be life-threatening. Immediate medical management is required to stabilize the patient. Early recognition significantly improves outcomes.

Q233. Answer: B

Explanation: Somatic symptom disorder involves excessive focus on physical symptoms that cause significant distress. Individuals may experience genuine bodily sensations but interpret them as severe illness. The preoccupation persists even when medical evaluation reveals minimal findings. Psychological factors often contribute to the severity of concern. The condition can lead to frequent healthcare visits and impaired functioning. Treatment focuses on supportive care and psychological therapy.

Q234. Answer: A

Explanation: Disruptive mood dysregulation disorder involves chronic irritability and severe recurrent temper outbursts. The symptoms typically begin during childhood and occur in multiple settings. Outbursts are disproportionate to the situation and inconsistent with developmental level. Between episodes, the individual often remains persistently irritable or angry. The disorder was introduced to reduce overdiagnosis of pediatric bipolar disorder. Treatment often includes behavioral interventions and psychotherapy.

Q235. Answer: C

Explanation: Trichotillomania is characterized by recurrent hair pulling that results in hair loss. Individuals often experience increasing tension before pulling and relief afterward. The behavior may occur automatically or in response to stress. Over time it can lead to significant cosmetic and emotional distress. The condition is classified among obsessive-compulsive related disorders. Behavioral therapy is often an effective treatment approach.

Q236. Answer: C

Explanation: Intermittent explosive disorder involves recurrent impulsive outbursts of aggression. These episodes are disproportionate to the triggering event. The behavior may include verbal aggression or physical acts toward people or property. Individuals often report feeling relief after the outburst but later experience regret. The disorder can significantly disrupt social and occupational functioning. Treatment may involve psychotherapy and medication to improve impulse control.

Q237. Answer: D

Explanation: Narcolepsy is a sleep disorder characterized by excessive daytime sleepiness and sudden sleep attacks. Many individuals also experience sleep paralysis during transitions between sleep and wakefulness. During these episodes, the person is conscious but temporarily unable to move. Additional features may include vivid dream-like hallucinations and sudden muscle weakness. The disorder involves dysregulation of sleep-wake cycles in the brain. Treatment focuses on improving alertness and regulating sleep patterns.

Q238. Answer: B

Explanation: Antisocial personality disorder involves a pervasive disregard for the rights of others. Individuals may engage in deceitful, manipulative, or unlawful behavior. Lack of remorse after harming others is a common characteristic. These traits typically begin in adolescence and continue into adulthood. Impulsivity and irresponsibility frequently accompany the behavior pattern. Long-term therapeutic engagement may help manage associated problems.

Q239. Answer: C

Explanation: Insomnia disorder involves difficulty initiating or maintaining sleep despite adequate opportunity. Individuals often experience fatigue, irritability, and impaired daytime functioning. Stress, medical conditions, or psychological factors may contribute to the problem. Chronic insomnia can significantly affect overall health and quality of life. Behavioral sleep interventions are often effective treatments. Medication may be considered when symptoms persist.

Q240. Answer: B

Explanation: Separation anxiety disorder involves excessive fear or distress related to separation from attachment figures. Although commonly diagnosed in children, it may also occur in adults. Individuals worry excessively about harm coming to loved ones or about being abandoned. The anxiety can lead to avoidance of situations that require separation. Symptoms often interfere with social, academic, or occupational functioning. Treatment typically includes psychotherapy and supportive interventions.

Q241. Answer: B

Explanation: Somatic symptom disorder involves persistent concern about physical symptoms that cause significant distress and impairment. The symptoms may or may not have a clear medical explanation. Individuals often experience intense anxiety about their health and may frequently seek medical care. The focus is on the disproportionate thoughts and behaviors related to the symptoms rather than the symptoms themselves. This pattern often leads to repeated medical evaluations and frustration when tests are normal. Psychological interventions can help individuals manage distress and improve functioning.

Q242. Answer: A

Explanation: Conversion disorder involves neurological symptoms that cannot be explained by underlying medical conditions. These symptoms often arise following psychological stress or trauma. Individuals may experience paralysis, blindness, or seizures without physiological evidence of disease. The symptoms are not intentionally produced and can cause significant distress or functional impairment. Psychological factors are believed to influence the development of the condition. Treatment often involves psychotherapy and supportive care.

Q243. Answer: B

Explanation: Factitious disorder involves the intentional production or exaggeration of physical or psychological symptoms. The motivation is to assume the role of a patient rather than obtain external rewards. Individuals may falsify medical history or even induce symptoms to receive medical attention. The behavior occurs in the absence of obvious incentives such as financial gain. This condition can lead to unnecessary medical procedures and significant healthcare utilization. Management requires careful psychiatric assessment and supportive therapeutic strategies.

Q244. Answer: A

Explanation: Illness anxiety disorder is characterized by excessive worry about having or developing a serious illness. Individuals often misinterpret normal bodily sensations as signs of severe disease. Medical evaluations typically reveal little or no pathology. Despite reassurance from healthcare providers, the anxiety persists. The preoccupation can significantly interfere with daily life. Treatment usually focuses on cognitive behavioral therapy and anxiety management strategies.

Q245. Answer: B

Explanation: Brief psychotic disorder involves the sudden onset of psychotic symptoms such as hallucinations, delusions, or disorganized speech. The episode lasts at least one day but less than one month. Symptoms often occur following a significant stressor or traumatic event. Individuals usually return to their previous level of functioning after recovery. Early recognition is important for ensuring patient safety and providing supportive treatment. Short-term antipsychotic medication may sometimes be required.

Q246. Answer: D

Explanation: Schizophrenia is a chronic psychiatric disorder characterized by psychotic symptoms lasting longer than six months. These symptoms may include hallucinations, delusions, disorganized speech, and impaired functioning. Negative symptoms such as social withdrawal and reduced emotional expression are also common. The disorder significantly affects occupational and social functioning. Early treatment improves long-term outcomes and quality of life. Management typically involves antipsychotic medications and psychosocial support.

Q247. Answer: B

Explanation: Cyclothymic disorder involves chronic mood fluctuations including periods of hypomanic symptoms and mild depressive symptoms. These episodes do not meet full criteria for manic or major depressive episodes. The pattern persists for at least two years in adults. Individuals may appear emotionally unstable or unpredictable. Although symptoms may be less severe, they can still interfere with daily functioning. Long-term monitoring and supportive therapy are often recommended.

Q248. Answer: D

Explanation: Bipolar II disorder involves a pattern of recurrent major depressive episodes and hypomanic episodes. Hypomania is similar to mania but less severe and does not cause significant functional impairment. Individuals with this disorder never experience a full manic episode. Depressive episodes are often more frequent and disabling. Accurate diagnosis is important because treatment strategies differ from those used for unipolar depression. Mood stabilizers and psychotherapy are commonly used treatments.

Q249. Answer: A

Explanation: Intrusive thoughts are unwanted and distressing thoughts that enter consciousness repeatedly. They often occur in obsessive-compulsive disorder and can involve themes that conflict with personal values. The individual recognizes that the thoughts are irrational but finds them difficult to dismiss. These thoughts may cause significant anxiety and distress. Compulsive behaviors are sometimes performed to neutralize the anxiety associated with them. Cognitive behavioral therapy helps individuals learn strategies to manage these experiences.

Q250. Answer: A

Explanation: Specific phobia involves intense fear of a particular object or situation. The fear is excessive compared with the actual danger posed. Individuals often go to great lengths to avoid the feared stimulus. Exposure to the trigger typically produces immediate anxiety. Although the person may recognize the fear as unreasonable, avoidance behaviors persist. Behavioral therapies such as exposure therapy are effective treatments.

Q251. Answer: D

Explanation: Agoraphobia involves fear or anxiety related to situations where escape may be difficult or help may not be available. Common triggers include crowded places, public transportation, or being outside the home alone. Individuals may avoid these situations or endure them with extreme distress. The condition frequently develops in association with panic disorder. Avoidance behaviors can lead to severe social isolation. Treatment often involves cognitive behavioral therapy and gradual exposure techniques.

Q252. Answer: B

Explanation: Binge eating disorder involves recurrent episodes of consuming large amounts of food within a short period. Individuals often feel a loss of control during these episodes. Unlike bulimia nervosa, compensatory behaviors such as vomiting or laxative use are absent. The disorder may lead to weight gain and emotional distress. Feelings of shame or guilt commonly follow binge episodes. Treatment may include psychotherapy, nutritional counseling, and behavioral interventions.

Q253. Answer: D

Explanation: Individuals with anorexia nervosa often have a severely distorted perception of their body weight or shape. Even when dangerously underweight, they may believe they are overweight. This cognitive distortion contributes to restrictive eating behaviors and extreme weight loss. The disorder carries significant medical risks including cardiovascular complications and malnutrition. Psychological factors and sociocultural influences often play a role in its development. Early treatment improves prognosis and reduces long-term complications.

Q254. Answer: B

Explanation: Excoriation disorder involves recurrent skin picking that leads to tissue damage. Individuals may attempt to stop the behavior but often find it difficult to control. The behavior may occur in response to stress, anxiety, or boredom. Over time, repeated picking can lead to infections and scarring. The disorder belongs to the obsessive-compulsive related disorders category. Behavioral therapies are commonly used in treatment.

Q255. Answer: B

Explanation: Dependent personality disorder is characterized by a pervasive need to be cared for by others. Individuals often have difficulty making everyday decisions without excessive advice or reassurance. They may feel helpless when alone and fear abandonment. This dependency can lead to submissive or clingy behavior in relationships. The pattern typically begins in early adulthood and affects many aspects of life. Psychotherapy may help individuals develop greater independence and self-confidence.

Q256. Answer: A

Explanation: Avoidant personality disorder involves a pervasive pattern of social inhibition and feelings of inadequacy. Individuals are extremely sensitive to criticism or rejection. They may desire social relationships but avoid interactions due to fear of embarrassment. This avoidance often leads to isolation and limited social experiences. The condition can significantly affect occupational and interpersonal functioning. Therapeutic interventions focus on building confidence and improving social skills.

Q257. Answer: B

Explanation: Schizoid personality disorder is characterized by detachment from social relationships and restricted emotional expression. Individuals often prefer solitary activities and appear indifferent to praise or criticism. They typically show little desire for close relationships. Emotional responses may appear flat or limited. Although functioning may remain stable, interpersonal connections are minimal. Treatment focuses on improving social functioning when the individual seeks help.

Q258. Answer: A

Explanation: Schizotypal personality disorder involves social deficits along with cognitive or perceptual distortions. Individuals may hold unusual beliefs or experience magical thinking. Their behavior and appearance may seem eccentric or odd to others. They often experience discomfort in close relationships. Although reality testing remains mostly intact, thinking patterns may resemble mild psychotic features. Psychotherapy can help improve social functioning and coping strategies.

Q259. Answer: D

Explanation: Paranoid personality disorder is characterized by pervasive distrust and suspicion of others. Individuals often interpret neutral events as threatening or malicious. They may hold grudges and be reluctant to confide in others. This persistent mistrust can interfere with social and occupational relationships. The behavior pattern usually begins by early adulthood. Therapeutic engagement requires patience and careful development of trust.

Q260. Answer: A

Explanation: Borderline personality disorder involves instability in interpersonal relationships, self-image, and emotional regulation. Individuals may experience intense mood swings and chronic feelings of emptiness. Fear of abandonment often leads to frantic efforts to avoid real or perceived rejection. Impulsive behaviors such as self-harm or risky activities may occur. Relationships frequently alternate between extremes of idealization and devaluation. Dialectical behavior therapy is a commonly used treatment approach.

Q261. Answer: D

Explanation: Loose associations refer to a disturbance in the logical connection between thoughts. Speech may shift from one topic to another with little or no meaningful relationship between ideas. This pattern is commonly observed in psychotic disorders. The individual may appear incoherent or difficult to follow during conversation. It reflects disruption in normal thought organization and cognitive processing. Assessment of thought processes is an essential component of the mental status examination.

Q262. Answer: D

Explanation: Akathisia is a movement disorder commonly associated with antipsychotic medications. It is characterized by subjective feelings of inner restlessness accompanied by constant movement. Patients may pace, shift weight frequently, or feel unable to sit still. The condition results from dopamine blockade in motor pathways of the brain. Symptoms can be very distressing and may lead to nonadherence with treatment. Management may include dose adjustment or additional medications to relieve symptoms.

Q263. Answer: D

Explanation: Tardive dyskinesia is a late-onset movement disorder associated with prolonged use of dopamine-blocking medications. It typically presents with repetitive, involuntary movements of the face, tongue, and mouth. These movements may include lip smacking, grimacing, or tongue protrusion. The condition may become irreversible if not recognized early. Regular monitoring for abnormal movements is recommended for patients receiving long-term antipsychotic therapy. Adjusting medication may help reduce progression of symptoms.

Q264. Answer: D

Explanation: Command hallucinations involve auditory hallucinations that direct an individual to perform specific actions. The voices may instruct harmless behaviors or potentially dangerous activities. These hallucinations are particularly concerning because they may increase the risk of harm. Assessment should evaluate the patient's willingness to act on the commands. Immediate safety evaluation is essential in such situations. Antipsychotic medications and supportive interventions are commonly used in treatment.

Q265. Answer: B

Explanation: Thought blocking refers to an abrupt interruption in the flow of thought. The individual may suddenly stop speaking and appear unable to continue the conversation. After a pause, they may start a completely new topic. This phenomenon is often observed in psychotic disorders. It reflects disruption in normal cognitive processing. Clinicians assess the frequency and context of these episodes during mental status examinations.

Q266. Answer: B

Explanation: Neologisms are newly created words or phrases that are not recognized within standard language. These words typically have meaning only to the individual who uses them. This speech abnormality is frequently associated with schizophrenia. It reflects a disturbance in language organization and thought processes. The presence of neologisms may make communication difficult. Careful observation of speech patterns assists in accurate psychiatric assessment.

Q267. Answer: B

Explanation: Perseveration refers to the persistent repetition of a particular word, phrase, or idea. The individual continues to focus on the same response even when the conversation changes. This behavior may occur in several psychiatric or neurological conditions. It indicates difficulty shifting cognitive focus. Observing this pattern can provide insight into underlying cognitive dysfunction. Mental status examination includes evaluating such disturbances in thought processes.

Q268. Answer: A

Explanation: Specific phobia involves intense and irrational fear of a particular object or situation. Exposure to the feared stimulus often produces immediate anxiety or panic. Individuals frequently avoid the trigger to prevent distress. Although the fear may be recognized as excessive, it remains difficult to control. The condition can significantly interfere with daily activities. Behavioral therapies, particularly exposure-based interventions, are effective treatments.

Q269. Answer: A

Explanation: Sleep-related eating disorder involves episodes of eating during partial arousal from sleep. Individuals often have little or no memory of the behavior the next day. The condition is classified among sleep disorders rather than eating disorders. Episodes typically occur during non-REM sleep stages. The behavior can lead to weight gain and safety risks if dangerous items are consumed. Management may involve addressing underlying sleep disturbances.

Q270. Answer: C

Explanation: Histrionic personality disorder involves excessive emotionality and attention-seeking behavior. Individuals often display dramatic and theatrical emotional expressions. They may exaggerate situations to maintain attention from others. Relationships can appear superficial or rapidly shifting. The behavior pattern usually begins in early adulthood. Psychotherapy can help individuals develop healthier interpersonal relationships.

Q271. Answer: A

Explanation: Narcissistic personality disorder is characterized by grandiosity and a strong need for admiration. Individuals often believe they are superior to others and expect special treatment. They may have difficulty empathizing with the feelings of others. Criticism can provoke strong defensive reactions. Relationships may be strained due to exploitative or self-centered behavior. Psychotherapeutic approaches focus on developing empathy and realistic self-perception.

Q272. Answer: C

Explanation: Borderline personality disorder involves instability in mood, relationships, and self-image. Individuals often experience rapid emotional changes and intense anger. Impulsive behaviors such as self-harm or substance use may occur. Fear of abandonment frequently influences interpersonal interactions. Relationships may alternate between extreme closeness and hostility. Structured psychotherapy is often effective in managing symptoms.

Q273. Answer: C

Explanation: Obsessive-compulsive disorder involves intrusive thoughts known as obsessions and repetitive behaviors called compulsions. Obsessions create significant anxiety and distress. Compulsions are performed to neutralize these thoughts or reduce anxiety. The behaviors can become time-consuming and interfere with daily functioning. Neurobiological studies suggest involvement of specific brain circuits regulating behavior. Treatment commonly includes psychotherapy and medication.

Q274. Answer: A

Explanation: Post-traumatic stress disorder develops after exposure to a traumatic event. Individuals may experience intrusive memories, hypervigilance, and difficulty concentrating. Emotional numbness and avoidance of reminders of the trauma are also common. Symptoms typically persist for more than one month. The disorder can significantly impair functioning and quality of life. Trauma-focused psychotherapy is an important component of treatment.

Q275. Answer: D

Explanation: Major depressive disorder involves a sustained period of depressed mood or loss of interest in activities. Symptoms must persist for at least two weeks and cause significant impairment. Additional features may include fatigue, sleep disturbances, and changes in appetite. Cognitive symptoms such as feelings of worthlessness or difficulty concentrating may occur. The condition can affect emotional, physical, and social functioning. Effective treatments include psychotherapy and antidepressant medications.

Q276. Answer: A

Explanation: Mania is a state of abnormally elevated or irritable mood accompanied by increased activity or energy. Symptoms include decreased need for sleep, grandiosity, rapid speech, and impulsive behavior. Episodes typically last at least one week or require hospitalization. The condition may lead to risky decision-making and impaired judgment. Mania significantly disrupts social and occupational functioning. Mood stabilizing medications are commonly used in treatment.

Q277. Answer: C

Explanation: Medical conditions such as thyroid disorders can produce symptoms that resemble psychiatric disorders. Hypothyroidism often causes fatigue, low mood, and cognitive slowing. Recognizing underlying medical causes is essential before diagnosing a primary psychiatric disorder. Treatment of the medical condition often improves psychological symptoms. Comprehensive assessment includes laboratory evaluation when appropriate. Integration of medical and psychiatric care improves patient outcomes.

Q278. Answer: C

Explanation: Body dysmorphic disorder involves excessive concern with perceived flaws in physical appearance. These perceived defects are usually minor or not observable to others. Individuals may become preoccupied with specific body parts or characteristics. The concern often leads to repetitive checking behaviors or attempts to hide the perceived defect. Social functioning may be impaired due to embarrassment or shame. Treatment commonly includes psychotherapy and medication.

Q279. Answer: D

Explanation: Attention-deficit hyperactivity disorder involves persistent patterns of inattention and hyperactivity. Symptoms often appear during childhood and may continue into adulthood. Individuals may struggle with organization, impulsivity, and sustaining attention. Academic and occupational functioning may be affected. The disorder is associated with differences in brain development and neurotransmitter activity. Treatment may include behavioral interventions and medication.

Q280. Answer: A

Explanation: Antisocial personality disorder involves a persistent pattern of disregard for social norms and the rights of others. Individuals may engage in deceitful, manipulative, or criminal behavior. Lack of remorse after harming others is a defining characteristic. Impulsivity and irresponsibility frequently accompany this pattern. The behavior typically begins during adolescence and continues into adulthood. Long-term treatment focuses on behavioral management and improving social functioning.

Q281. Answer: C

Explanation: Parasomnias involve abnormal behaviors occurring during sleep or transitions between sleep stages. Sleepwalking is a common example and occurs during deep non-REM sleep. Individuals may walk, talk, or perform routine actions without awareness. Episodes typically occur in the first third of the night. Most individuals have little memory of the event afterward. Management focuses on ensuring safety and addressing contributing sleep factors.

Q282. Answer: D

Explanation: Generalized anxiety disorder involves excessive and uncontrollable worry about multiple aspects of life. The anxiety occurs most days for at least six months. Individuals often experience physical symptoms such as muscle tension and fatigue. The constant worry interferes with daily functioning and concentration. Emotional distress may affect relationships and work performance. Treatment commonly includes psychotherapy and medication.

Q283. Answer: C

Explanation: Substance-induced psychotic disorder occurs when hallucinations or delusions develop during or soon after substance intoxication or withdrawal. Certain drugs can disrupt neurotransmitter systems and alter perception. Symptoms typically improve after the substance is cleared from the body. Careful assessment is required to distinguish this condition from primary psychotic disorders. Treatment focuses on stabilization and substance use management. Long-term prognosis depends on abstinence and supportive care.

Q284. Answer: B

Explanation: Hypnagogic hallucinations occur during the transition from wakefulness to sleep. These experiences may involve vivid visual or auditory sensations. They are commonly associated with sleep disorders such as narcolepsy but can occur in healthy individuals as well. The person typically recognizes the experience as dreamlike after awakening. Although often benign, frequent episodes may warrant further evaluation. Understanding sleep-related hallucinations helps prevent misdiagnosis.

Q285. Answer: A

Explanation: Hypnopompic hallucinations occur during the transition from sleep to wakefulness. These experiences may involve vivid sensory perceptions such as voices or images. They can be frightening but are usually brief and harmless. Such hallucinations are often associated with narcolepsy or sleep deprivation. They differ from psychotic hallucinations because they occur in relation to sleep states. Education and reassurance may help reduce anxiety related to these episodes.

Q286. Answer: A

Explanation: A delusion of reference involves the belief that ordinary events or messages have special personal meaning. Individuals may interpret media broadcasts or conversations as directed specifically toward them. This misinterpretation occurs despite lack of evidence. The belief remains fixed even when logical explanations are offered. Such delusions are often associated with psychotic disorders. Treatment typically involves antipsychotic medication and supportive therapy.

Q287. Answer: B

Explanation: Grandiose delusions involve exaggerated beliefs about one's importance, abilities, or identity. Individuals may believe they possess exceptional talents or a special mission. These beliefs are firmly held despite contradictory evidence. Grandiosity can occur in manic episodes or psychotic disorders. The symptom may lead to unrealistic decisions or risky behaviors. Treatment focuses on stabilizing mood and reducing psychotic symptoms.

Q288. Answer: D

Explanation: Delusions of persecution involve the belief that one is being targeted, harmed, or conspired against. Individuals may feel constantly threatened by others. These beliefs are resistant to logical argument or contradictory information. The symptom is commonly associated with psychotic disorders such as schizophrenia. It can significantly impair trust and social functioning. Antipsychotic treatment and supportive care help manage these symptoms.

Q289. Answer: B

Explanation: Nihilistic delusions involve the belief that parts of the body, the self, or the world no longer exist or have ceased functioning. These beliefs may include ideas of being dead or having no organs. The symptom is rare but may occur in severe depressive or psychotic states. It reflects profound disturbance in perception of reality. The experience can cause extreme distress and functional impairment. Treatment typically requires intensive psychiatric care.

Q290. Answer: C
Explanation: Fear of heights is a common form of specific phobia. Individuals experience intense anxiety when confronted with the feared situation. Avoidance behavior often develops to prevent exposure. The fear is disproportionate to the actual danger posed. Despite recognizing the irrational nature of the fear, the person finds it difficult to control the response. Behavioral exposure therapy is highly effective in treatment.
Q291. Answer: D
Explanation: Auditory hallucinations involve perceiving sounds without an external stimulus. These sounds may include voices, music, or environmental noises. The experience can feel very real to the individual. Such hallucinations may occur in psychotic disorders or neurological conditions. The severity and impact vary depending on the underlying cause. Treatment focuses on addressing the primary disorder responsible for the symptom.
Q292. Answer: C
Explanation: An illusion occurs when a real external stimulus is misinterpreted or perceived incorrectly. In this case, the coat is a real object but is mistaken for something else. Illusions are common in situations involving poor lighting or heightened emotional states. Unlike hallucinations, they involve actual sensory input. Understanding the difference between illusions and hallucinations is important during psychiatric assessment. Illusions may also occur in delirium or severe anxiety.
Q293. Answer: D
Explanation: Derealization involves a subjective sense that the external environment is strange or unreal. Individuals may describe the world as dreamlike or distorted. Although the experience is unsettling, the person usually recognizes that it is a perception rather than reality. Such symptoms can occur during severe anxiety, trauma, or dissociative disorders. Episodes may be temporary but distressing. Psychological treatment often focuses on stress reduction and grounding techniques.
Q294. Answer: C
Explanation: Depersonalization involves a sense of detachment from one's own body or mental processes. Individuals may feel as though they are observing themselves from an external perspective. The experience can occur during extreme stress or trauma. Despite the unusual sensation, reality testing remains intact. Episodes are often brief but may recur during anxiety disorders. Therapeutic approaches focus on reducing stress and improving emotional regulation.
Q295. Answer: C
Explanation: Mutism refers to the absence of speech despite intact ability to speak. It may occur in certain psychiatric conditions such as severe depression or psychotic disorders. Some individuals exhibit selective mutism in specific social situations. The behavior can also be associated with trauma or anxiety. Assessment should evaluate psychological and environmental factors contributing to the condition. Treatment strategies depend on the underlying cause.
Q296. Answer: A
Explanation: Catatonia is a psychomotor syndrome characterized by abnormal movement patterns and behavioral abnormalities. Individuals may remain motionless or maintain unusual postures for extended periods. Resistance to movement by others may also occur. The condition can appear in mood disorders, psychotic disorders, or medical conditions. Prompt recognition is important because it can respond well to specific treatments. Early intervention improves outcomes and prevents complications.
Q297. Answer: A
Explanation: Flight of ideas involves rapid shifting between topics with superficial associations. The speech may appear pressured and difficult to interrupt. This pattern is commonly observed during manic episodes. Although connections between ideas exist, they are often loosely related. The rapid pace can make communication challenging. Stabilizing mood symptoms often reduces this speech disturbance.
Q298. Answer: B

Explanation: Tangential speech occurs when responses diverge from the topic and never return to the original question. The individual's answers may be loosely related but fail to address what was asked. This pattern reflects disorganized thinking. It is frequently observed in psychotic disorders. Careful questioning during mental status examination helps identify this disturbance. Treatment focuses on managing the underlying psychiatric condition.

Q299. Answer: C

Explanation: Narcissistic personality disorder involves grandiosity and a strong need for admiration. Individuals often view themselves as superior to others. They may expect preferential treatment and become angry when their expectations are not met. Empathy for others may be limited. Relationships may become strained due to exploitative behaviors. Psychotherapy focuses on improving interpersonal awareness and emotional regulation.

Q300. Answer: C

Explanation: Delirium is an acute disturbance in attention and awareness that develops over a short period. The condition is often caused by medical illness, infection, or medication effects. Individuals may experience confusion, disorientation, and fluctuating levels of consciousness. Symptoms often worsen during the evening or night. Early recognition is essential because delirium may indicate a serious underlying medical problem. Treatment focuses on addressing the underlying cause and providing supportive care.

Question (301-400)

Q301. A patient taking a monoamine oxidase inhibitor consumes aged cheese and develops severe headache, hypertension, and palpitations. What is the most likely cause of this reaction?

(A) Serotonin depletion
(B) Dopamine receptor blockade
(C) Tyramine accumulation causing catecholamine release
(D) Cholinergic overstimulation

Q302. A patient with major depressive disorder reports persistent sadness, loss of interest in hobbies, and fatigue for the past month. Which neurotransmitter deficiency is most strongly linked with these symptoms?

(A) Serotonin
(B) Dopamine
(C) Histamine
(D) Acetylcholine

Q303. A patient taking lithium presents with tremor, diarrhea, confusion, and unsteady gait. What should the nurse practitioner suspect?

(A) Lithium toxicity
(B) Neuroleptic malignant syndrome
(C) Serotonin syndrome
(D) Anticholinergic toxicity

Q304. Which symptom is most characteristic of generalized anxiety disorder?

(A) Fear of social scrutiny and embarrassment
(B) Recurrent intrusive thoughts with compulsive rituals
(C) Persistent and excessive worry about multiple aspects of life
(D) Sudden episodes of intense fear with palpitations

Q305. A patient reports hearing voices that comment on their actions when no one else is present. What type of symptom does this represent?

(A) Compulsion
(B) Hallucination
(C) Illusion
(D) Delusion

Q306. A patient treated with haloperidol develops muscle rigidity, fever, autonomic instability, and altered consciousness. What is the most likely diagnosis?

(A) Acute dystonia
(B) Neuroleptic malignant syndrome
(C) Akathisia
(D) Serotonin syndrome

Q307. A patient states, "The government placed a chip in my brain to control my thoughts." What psychiatric symptom is demonstrated?

(A) Nihilistic delusion
(B) Persecutory delusion
(C) Grandiose delusion
(D) Somatic delusion

Q308. A patient with bipolar disorder presents with elevated mood, decreased need for sleep, pressured speech, and increased goal-directed activity lasting one week. What episode is most consistent with these findings?

(A) Manic episode

(B) Hypomanic episode
(C) Cyclothymic episode
(D) Major depressive episode

Q309. A patient experiences recurrent intrusive thoughts about contamination and repeatedly washes their hands for hours each day. What disorder is most consistent with these symptoms?
(A) Illness anxiety disorder
(B) Panic disorder
(C) Obsessive-compulsive disorder
(D) Generalized anxiety disorder

Q310. A patient taking clozapine requires regular blood monitoring due to the risk of which serious adverse effect?
(A) Pulmonary embolism
(B) Hepatic failure
(C) Agranulocytosis
(D) Renal toxicity

Q311. A patient demonstrates repetitive, purposeless motor movements such as pacing and inability to remain still after starting an antipsychotic. What condition is most likely present?
(A) Parkinsonism
(B) Akathisia
(C) Tardive dyskinesia
(D) Dystonia

Q312. A child repeatedly loses temper, argues with adults, and deliberately annoys others for at least six months. What disorder is most consistent with these behaviors?
(A) Intermittent explosive disorder
(B) Attention-deficit hyperactivity disorder
(C) Oppositional defiant disorder
(D) Conduct disorder

Q313. Which defense mechanism involves refusing to acknowledge an unpleasant reality or emotion?
(A) Denial
(B) Displacement
(C) Projection
(D) Sublimation

Q314. A patient suddenly develops painful muscle spasms of the neck and jaw shortly after receiving an antipsychotic medication. What is the most likely cause?
(A) Parkinsonism
(B) Acute dystonia
(C) Akathisia
(D) Tardive dyskinesia

Q315. A patient describes feeling detached from their own body and perceives themselves as observing their actions from outside. What phenomenon is this?
(A) Derealization
(B) Dissociation
(C) Delusion
(D) Depersonalization

Q316. A patient taking selective serotonin reuptake inhibitors develops agitation, hyperreflexia, sweating, and tremor after starting another serotonergic medication. What condition should be suspected?
(A) Neuroleptic malignant syndrome

(B) Serotonin syndrome
(C) Lithium toxicity
(D) Anticholinergic toxicity

Q317. Which neurotransmitter is primarily associated with reward, motivation, and pleasure pathways in the brain?

(A) Dopamine
(B) Glutamate
(C) Acetylcholine
(D) GABA

Q318. A patient persistently lies, steals, and shows lack of remorse for harming others beginning in adolescence. What diagnosis is most consistent with this pattern in adulthood?

(A) Histrionic personality disorder
(B) Antisocial personality disorder
(C) Borderline personality disorder
(D) Narcissistic personality disorder

Q319. A patient experiences sudden episodes of intense fear accompanied by chest pain, dizziness, and shortness of breath that peak within minutes. What disorder is most likely?

(A) Panic disorder
(B) Agoraphobia
(C) Social anxiety disorder
(D) Specific phobia

Q320. A patient repeatedly checks the stove dozens of times before leaving the house despite knowing it is already turned off. What psychological process maintains this behavior?

(A) Punishment
(B) Positive reinforcement
(C) Negative reinforcement
(D) Extinction

Q321. A patient with schizophrenia shows diminished emotional expression, reduced speech output, and lack of motivation. These symptoms are classified as what type?

(A) Positive symptoms
(B) Cognitive symptoms
(C) Mood symptoms
(D) Negative symptoms

Q322. A patient reports a persistent pattern of unstable relationships, impulsivity, fear of abandonment, and intense mood swings. Which disorder is most consistent with these features?

(A) Schizoid personality disorder
(B) Avoidant personality disorder
(C) Borderline personality disorder
(D) Dependent personality disorder

Q323. A patient with depression begins treatment with an SSRI and reports improved mood after several weeks. What mechanism best explains this therapeutic effect?

(A) Gradual neuroadaptive changes in serotonergic pathways
(B) Immediate receptor blockade
(C) Dopamine receptor stimulation
(D) Increased acetylcholine release

Q324. A patient believes that strangers on television are sending secret messages directly to them. What type of delusion is this?

(A) Nihilistic delusion

(B) Delusion of reference
(C) Delusion of grandeur
(D) Somatic delusion

Q325. A patient reports persistent fear of being judged or embarrassed in social situations such as public speaking or meeting unfamiliar people. What disorder best explains these symptoms?
(A) Panic disorder
(B) Generalized anxiety disorder
(C) Specific phobia
(D) Social anxiety disorder

Q326. A patient receiving long-term antipsychotic therapy develops involuntary facial movements, lip smacking, and tongue protrusion. What disorder is most likely present?
(A) Akathisia
(B) Parkinsonism
(C) Acute dystonia
(D) Tardive dyskinesia

Q327. A patient reports difficulty concentrating, fatigue, and irritability after experiencing prolonged stress at work. What physiological system is primarily activated during chronic stress?
(A) Somatic nervous system
(B) Enteric nervous system
(C) Hypothalamic-pituitary-adrenal axis
(D) Parasympathetic nervous system

Q328. A patient presents with sudden memory loss for personal information after experiencing a traumatic event but remains otherwise alert. What condition is most consistent with this presentation?
(A) Dissociative amnesia
(B) Delirium
(C) Factitious disorder
(D) Alzheimer disease

Q329. A patient reports persistently elevated self-importance, fantasies of unlimited success, and a need for excessive admiration. Which personality disorder best fits this description?
(A) Narcissistic personality disorder
(B) Borderline personality disorder
(C) Avoidant personality disorder
(D) Dependent personality disorder

Q330. A patient with depression reports sleeping excessively and experiencing increased appetite and weight gain. What subtype of depression includes these features?
(A) Seasonal features
(B) Psychotic features
(C) Melancholic features
(D) Atypical features

Q331. A patient describes persistent fear of flying and avoids air travel whenever possible. What classification best describes this condition?
(A) Social anxiety disorder
(B) Generalized anxiety disorder
(C) Specific phobia
(D) Panic disorder

Q332. A patient with schizophrenia demonstrates disorganized speech with frequent derailment and illogical connections between ideas. What thought process disturbance is illustrated?
(A) Loose associations

(B) Circumstantiality
(C) Flight of ideas
(D) Perseveration

Q333. A patient frequently expresses excessive concern about having a serious illness despite repeated negative medical tests. What disorder is most consistent with this pattern?
(A) Conversion disorder
(B) Somatic symptom disorder
(C) Illness anxiety disorder
(D) Factitious disorder

Q334. A patient reports feeling emotionally numb and detached from their surroundings during a stressful event. Objects appear unreal or dreamlike. What experience is described?
(A) Dissociative identity disorder
(B) Delusional perception
(C) Depersonalization
(D) Derealization

Q335. A patient begins taking benzodiazepines for severe anxiety. What is the primary neurotransmitter system affected by these medications?
(A) Cholinergic system
(B) GABAergic system
(C) Serotonergic system
(D) Dopaminergic system

Q336. A patient who recently experienced trauma reports recurrent nightmares, hypervigilance, and avoidance of reminders of the event for several months. What disorder is most consistent with these symptoms?
(A) Acute stress disorder
(B) Posttraumatic stress disorder
(C) Panic disorder
(D) Adjustment disorder

Q337. A patient with bipolar disorder is prescribed valproate. What is the primary therapeutic purpose of this medication in this condition?
(A) Stimulate acetylcholine receptors
(B) Stabilize mood and reduce manic symptoms
(C) Increase dopamine release
(D) Enhance serotonin reuptake

Q338. A patient with severe depression reports persistent feelings of worthlessness and inappropriate guilt. These symptoms are most consistent with which diagnostic feature?
(A) Anxiety symptoms
(B) Somatic symptoms
(C) Cognitive symptoms of depression
(D) Psychotic symptoms

Q339. A patient shows limited emotional expression, prefers solitary activities, and appears indifferent to praise or criticism. What personality disorder best fits this description?
(A) Borderline personality disorder
(B) Schizoid personality disorder
(C) Histrionic personality disorder
(D) Narcissistic personality disorder

Q340. A patient experiences severe mood swings that correspond with seasonal changes, particularly worsening during winter months. What diagnosis should be considered?

(A) Persistent depressive disorder
(B) Bipolar disorder
(C) Cyclothymic disorder
(D) Major depressive disorder with seasonal pattern

Q341. A patient frequently exaggerates emotions, seeks constant attention, and behaves in a dramatic manner in social settings. Which personality disorder is most consistent with these behaviors?
(A) Dependent personality disorder
(B) Obsessive-compulsive personality disorder
(C) Avoidant personality disorder
(D) Histrionic personality disorder

Q342. A patient experiences chronic depressed mood for more than two years along with low energy and poor self-esteem. What condition best fits this description?
(A) Adjustment disorder
(B) Persistent depressive disorder
(C) Major depressive disorder
(D) Cyclothymic disorder

Q343. A patient displays rapid shifting of ideas, pressured speech, and jumping quickly from topic to topic while speaking. What thought pattern does this represent?
(A) Perseveration
(B) Tangential thinking
(C) Flight of ideas
(D) Thought blocking

Q344. A patient with severe anxiety begins practicing deep breathing and progressive muscle relaxation techniques. What therapeutic approach do these strategies represent?
(A) Humanistic therapy
(B) Behavioral therapy
(C) Interpersonal therapy
(D) Psychodynamic therapy

Q345. A patient reports hearing multiple voices arguing with each other about the patient's behavior. What type of hallucination is this?
(A) Auditory hallucination
(B) Tactile hallucination
(C) Visual hallucination
(D) Olfactory hallucination

Q346. A patient persistently organizes tasks with perfectionism and rigid adherence to rules, leading to difficulty completing projects. What personality disorder is most consistent with these characteristics?
(A) Avoidant personality disorder
(B) Narcissistic personality disorder
(C) Borderline personality disorder
(D) Obsessive-compulsive personality disorder

Q347. A patient states they feel constantly watched and monitored by unknown individuals despite lack of evidence. What symptom is illustrated?
(A) Illusion
(B) Paranoia
(C) Catatonia
(D) Compulsion

Q348. A patient experiencing opioid withdrawal reports muscle aches, sweating, nausea, and restlessness. What is the primary neurobiological cause of these symptoms?

(A) Increased serotonin release
(B) Enhanced acetylcholine transmission
(C) Excess dopamine activity
(D) Reduced endogenous opioid activity

Q349. A patient repeatedly fails to maintain employment and depends heavily on others to make everyday decisions. What personality disorder is most consistent with these behaviors?
(A) Dependent personality disorder
(B) Narcissistic personality disorder
(C) Paranoid personality disorder
(D) Schizotypal personality disorder

Q350. A patient believes that their organs are rotting and that they are already dead despite medical evidence proving otherwise. What type of delusion is this?
(A) Nihilistic delusion
(B) Grandiose delusion
(C) Somatic delusion
(D) Referential delusion

Q351. A patient with bipolar disorder reports a period of elevated mood lasting four days with increased energy, decreased need for sleep, and increased productivity but no major impairment in functioning. What episode is most consistent with these symptoms?
(A) Mixed episode
(B) Manic episode
(C) Hypomanic episode
(D) Cyclothymic episode

Q352. A patient repeatedly pulls out their hair, leading to noticeable hair loss and distress. What disorder is most consistent with this behavior?
(A) Body dysmorphic disorder
(B) Trichotillomania
(C) Excoriation disorder
(D) Somatic symptom disorder

Q353. A patient demonstrates persistent difficulty discarding possessions regardless of their value, leading to cluttered living spaces. What condition is most consistent with this behavior?
(A) Delusional disorder
(B) Schizotypal personality disorder
(C) Obsessive-compulsive disorder
(D) Hoarding disorder

Q354. A patient reports recurrent episodes of binge eating large amounts of food followed by self-induced vomiting. What eating disorder is most consistent with this pattern?
(A) Avoidant restrictive food intake disorder
(B) Bulimia nervosa
(C) Anorexia nervosa
(D) Binge eating disorder

Q355. A patient has persistent fear of leaving home alone or being in crowded places due to concern that escape may be difficult if panic occurs. What condition best explains these symptoms?
(A) Social anxiety disorder
(B) Specific phobia
(C) Panic disorder
(D) Agoraphobia

Q356. A patient suddenly stops speaking during a conversation and remains silent for several seconds before resuming. What thought disturbance is demonstrated?
(A) Neologism
(B) Tangentiality
(C) Circumstantiality
(D) Thought blocking
Q357. A patient presents with decreased facial expression, slowed movements, and rigidity after taking an antipsychotic medication. What adverse effect is most likely occurring?
(A) Tardive dyskinesia
(B) Acute dystonia
(C) Akathisia
(D) Parkinsonism
Q358. A patient with schizophrenia begins exhibiting rigid posture, minimal movement, and lack of response to external stimuli. What syndrome is most consistent with these findings?
(A) Catatonia
(B) Delirium
(C) Akathisia
(D) Dissociation
Q359. A patient repeatedly engages in skin picking that results in noticeable tissue damage. What disorder is most consistent with this behavior?
(A) Illness anxiety disorder
(B) Excoriation disorder
(C) Body dysmorphic disorder
(D) Somatic symptom disorder
Q360. A patient states that their thoughts are being broadcast to others through television signals. What psychotic symptom is illustrated?
(A) Thought insertion
(B) Delusion of reference
(C) Thought broadcasting
(D) Thought withdrawal
Q361. A patient with depression reports difficulty initiating activities and feeling unable to experience pleasure from normally enjoyable events. What symptom does this represent?
(A) Anhedonia
(B) Apathy
(C) Catatonia
(D) Dysphoria
Q362. A patient experiences recurrent episodes of eating large quantities of food but does not engage in compensatory behaviors afterward. What disorder best fits this pattern?
(A) Anorexia nervosa
(B) Binge eating disorder
(C) Bulimia nervosa
(D) Avoidant restrictive food intake disorder
Q363. A patient consistently avoids social relationships and feels inadequate in social situations due to fear of criticism or rejection. What personality disorder is most consistent with these behaviors?
(A) Narcissistic personality disorder
(B) Histrionic personality disorder
(C) Avoidant personality disorder
(D) Schizoid personality disorder

Q364. A patient reports persistent difficulty controlling anger and frequently engages in aggressive outbursts disproportionate to the situation. What disorder best explains this pattern?
(A) Antisocial personality disorder
(B) Conduct disorder
(C) Intermittent explosive disorder
(D) Oppositional defiant disorder
Q365. A patient with schizophrenia creates new words that have meaning only to them during conversation. What language disturbance is this called?
(A) Echolalia
(B) Neologism
(C) Perseveration
(D) Clang association
Q366. A patient reports that someone has placed thoughts into their mind that are not their own. What delusional experience does this represent?
(A) Thought broadcasting
(B) Delusion of reference
(C) Thought insertion
(D) Thought withdrawal
Q367. A patient is extremely preoccupied with a perceived flaw in their physical appearance that others barely notice. What disorder is most consistent with this concern?
(A) Somatic symptom disorder
(B) Delusional disorder
(C) Body dysmorphic disorder
(D) Illness anxiety disorder
Q368. A patient reports chronic feelings of emptiness and engages in impulsive behaviors such as reckless spending and substance use. What disorder is most consistent with these symptoms?
(A) Dependent personality disorder
(B) Narcissistic personality disorder
(C) Avoidant personality disorder
(D) Borderline personality disorder
Q369. A patient states that unrelated events such as conversations between strangers contain hidden messages directed specifically at them. What symptom is being demonstrated?
(A) Delusion of reference
(B) Grandiose delusion
(C) Somatic delusion
(D) Nihilistic delusion
Q370. A patient with severe depression experiences hallucinations and delusions that are consistent with their depressive mood. What diagnosis should be considered?
(A) Major depressive disorder with psychotic features
(B) Bipolar II disorder
(C) Cyclothymic disorder
(D) Persistent depressive disorder
Q371. A patient repeatedly imitates the words spoken by another person during conversation. What symptom is this called?
(A) Neologism
(B) Echolalia
(C) Perseveration
(D) Palilalia

Q372. A patient displays a persistent pattern of suspiciousness and distrust of others without sufficient basis. What personality disorder best fits this description?
(A) Avoidant personality disorder
(B) Dependent personality disorder
(C) Schizoid personality disorder
(D) Paranoid personality disorder
Q373. A patient exhibits exaggerated emotional expression and rapidly shifting moods during conversations. What personality disorder is most consistent with these traits?
(A) Histrionic personality disorder
(B) Borderline personality disorder
(C) Avoidant personality disorder
(D) Narcissistic personality disorder
Q374. A patient persistently believes they possess extraordinary abilities and superior intelligence compared with others. What type of delusion is this?
(A) Referential delusion
(B) Grandiose delusion
(C) Nihilistic delusion
(D) Persecutory delusion
Q375. A patient taking antipsychotic medication develops sustained upward deviation of the eyes. What movement disorder is most likely responsible?
(A) Oculogyric crisis
(B) Parkinsonism
(C) Tardive dyskinesia
(D) Akathisia
Q376. A patient reports persistent low mood and fatigue following a stressful life change but does not meet full criteria for major depression. What diagnosis should be considered?
(A) Bipolar disorder
(B) Cyclothymic disorder
(C) Persistent depressive disorder
(D) Adjustment disorder
Q377. A patient persistently neglects social norms, lies frequently, and shows little remorse for harmful actions. What personality disorder best explains these behaviors?
(A) Narcissistic personality disorder
(B) Antisocial personality disorder
(C) Avoidant personality disorder
(D) Borderline personality disorder
Q378. A patient experiences sudden confusion, disorientation, and fluctuating levels of consciousness over several hours. What condition is most likely present?
(A) Delirium
(B) Schizophrenia
(C) Dementia
(D) Dissociative disorder
Q379. A patient reports hearing voices that command them to perform certain actions. What type of hallucination is this?
(A) Olfactory hallucination
(B) Tactile hallucination
(C) Command hallucination
(D) Visual hallucination

Q380. A patient repeatedly returns to the same topic during conversation despite attempts to redirect the discussion. What speech pattern does this represent?
(A) Tangentiality
(B) Perseveration
(C) Flight of ideas
(D) Circumstantiality
Q381. A patient reports sudden episodes of intense fear accompanied by trembling, sweating, and feelings of impending doom. What type of episode is this?
(A) Panic attack
(B) Psychotic episode
(C) Dissociative episode
(D) Manic episode
Q382. A patient expresses excessive guilt and believes they deserve punishment for minor mistakes. What depressive symptom does this represent?
(A) Cognitive distortion
(B) Somatic complaint
(C) Psychomotor agitation
(D) Catatonic symptom
Q383. A patient shows limited interest in close relationships and prefers solitary activities without distress about being alone. What personality disorder is most consistent with this pattern?
(A) Schizoid personality disorder
(B) Borderline personality disorder
(C) Dependent personality disorder
(D) Avoidant personality disorder
Q384. A patient demonstrates rigid posture and maintains an unusual body position for extended periods without discomfort. What symptom is this?
(A) Waxy flexibility
(B) Akathisia
(C) Cataplexy
(D) Dystonia
Q385. A patient believes that their body emits a foul odor that others notice, although no odor is present. What type of delusion is this?
(A) Somatic delusion
(B) Nihilistic delusion
(C) Grandiose delusion
(D) Referential delusion
Q386. A patient develops agitation, tremor, and hyperthermia after combining two serotonergic medications. What condition should be suspected?
(A) Lithium toxicity
(B) Anticholinergic toxicity
(C) Serotonin syndrome
(D) Neuroleptic malignant syndrome
Q387. A patient frequently shifts from idealizing a person to suddenly devaluing them in relationships. What personality disorder is most consistent with this pattern?
(A) Schizoid personality disorder
(B) Narcissistic personality disorder
(C) Paranoid personality disorder
(D) Borderline personality disorder

Q388. A patient repeatedly washes hands for hours each day to relieve anxiety about contamination. What behavioral concept explains the continuation of this action?
(A) Positive reinforcement
(B) Negative reinforcement
(C) Extinction
(D) Punishment

Q389. A patient with bipolar disorder experiences depressive episodes alternating with periods of hypomania but never full mania. What diagnosis best fits this pattern?
(A) Persistent depressive disorder
(B) Bipolar I disorder
(C) Bipolar II disorder
(D) Cyclothymic disorder

Q390. A patient suddenly becomes mute and refuses to move despite being awake and aware. What syndrome is most consistent with these symptoms?
(A) Akathisia
(B) Dissociative fugue
(C) Delirium
(D) Catatonia

Q391. A patient persistently seeks reassurance and fears being abandoned if left alone. What personality disorder is most consistent with this behavior?
(A) Paranoid personality disorder
(B) Dependent personality disorder
(C) Narcissistic personality disorder
(D) Schizoid personality disorder

Q392. A patient repeatedly repeats their own words several times in succession during conversation. What speech abnormality is this?
(A) Palilalia
(B) Clang association
(C) Neologism
(D) Echolalia

Q393. A patient experiences persistent sadness, fatigue, and hopelessness lasting several weeks along with loss of interest in activities. What disorder is most consistent with these symptoms?
(A) Adjustment disorder
(B) Major depressive disorder
(C) Bipolar disorder
(D) Cyclothymic disorder

Q394. A patient believes that strangers are plotting to harm them despite evidence to the contrary. What type of delusion is this?
(A) Persecutory delusion
(B) Somatic delusion
(C) Referential delusion
(D) Grandiose delusion

Q395. A patient reports seeing insects crawling on the skin when none are present. What type of hallucination is this?
(A) Tactile hallucination
(B) Olfactory hallucination
(C) Gustatory hallucination
(D) Visual hallucination

Q396. A patient persistently exaggerates achievements and expects special treatment from others. What personality disorder best fits this behavior?

(A) Avoidant personality disorder

(B) Narcissistic personality disorder

(C) Dependent personality disorder

(D) Borderline personality disorder

Q397. A patient repeatedly organizes items symmetrically and becomes distressed if objects are slightly out of alignment. What disorder is most consistent with this behavior?

(A) Hoarding disorder

(B) Somatic symptom disorder

(C) Obsessive-compulsive disorder

(D) Body dysmorphic disorder

Q398. A patient suddenly travels away from home and cannot recall their personal identity afterward. What dissociative condition best explains this presentation?

(A) Dissociative amnesia

(B) Depersonalization disorder

(C) Conversion disorder

(D) Dissociative fugue

Q399. A patient expresses belief that their thoughts are being removed from their mind by an external force. What symptom is this called?

(A) Thought broadcasting

(B) Thought insertion

(C) Delusion of reference

(D) Thought withdrawal

Q400. A patient with depression begins experiencing significant improvement in mood and energy after several weeks of antidepressant therapy. What underlying process most likely explains this delayed improvement?

(A) Instant increase in dopamine release

(B) Direct stimulation of acetylcholine receptors

(C) Gradual neuroadaptive changes in brain signaling pathways

(D) Immediate neurotransmitter blockade

Answer Key and Explanation (301-400)

Q301. Answer: C

Explanation: Monoamine oxidase inhibitors block the enzyme responsible for breaking down monoamines such as tyramine. When foods rich in tyramine are consumed, tyramine accumulates and causes excessive release of norepinephrine from nerve terminals. This leads to sudden elevation in blood pressure, severe headache, and risk of hypertensive crisis. The reaction is known as the "cheese effect." It is a classic dietary interaction associated with this medication class. Avoidance of tyramine-containing foods is essential to prevent life-threatening complications.

Q302. Answer: A

Explanation: Serotonin is strongly associated with mood regulation, emotional stability, and feelings of well-being. Reduced serotonergic activity has been widely linked to depressive symptoms such as sadness, low motivation, and sleep disturbance. Many antidepressants work by increasing serotonin availability in the synaptic cleft. Selective serotonin reuptake inhibitors specifically target this neurotransmitter pathway. Restoration of serotonin transmission helps improve mood and emotional regulation. Dysregulation of this neurotransmitter is therefore a central feature in depressive disorders.

Q303. Answer: A

Explanation: Lithium toxicity occurs when serum lithium levels rise above the therapeutic range. Early symptoms include gastrointestinal distress, tremor, and weakness. As toxicity progresses, neurological manifestations such as confusion, ataxia, and seizures may develop. Lithium has a narrow therapeutic index, making monitoring essential. Factors such as dehydration, renal impairment, or drug interactions can increase lithium levels. Immediate evaluation of serum lithium concentration and supportive treatment are required.

Q304. Answer: C

Explanation: Generalized anxiety disorder is defined by chronic and excessive worry about a variety of everyday issues. Individuals often experience restlessness, fatigue, irritability, muscle tension, and difficulty concentrating. The worry is persistent and difficult to control for at least six months. It differs from panic disorder because symptoms are continuous rather than episodic. The anxiety also extends across multiple life domains rather than being limited to specific situations. This pervasive worry is the core diagnostic feature of the disorder.

Q305. Answer: B

Explanation: Hallucinations are perceptions that occur in the absence of an external stimulus. Auditory hallucinations are the most common type in psychotic disorders. Individuals may hear voices conversing, commenting, or giving commands. These experiences are perceived as real even though no external source exists. Hallucinations differ from illusions, which involve misinterpretation of real stimuli. Persistent hallucinations are frequently associated with schizophrenia and other psychotic conditions.

Q306. Answer: B

Explanation: Neuroleptic malignant syndrome is a rare but life-threatening reaction to antipsychotic medications. It is characterized by severe muscle rigidity, hyperthermia, autonomic instability, and altered mental status. The condition results from dopamine blockade in the central nervous system. Laboratory findings often include elevated creatine kinase due to muscle breakdown. Immediate discontinuation of the offending medication is required. Supportive care and medications such as dantrolene or bromocriptine may be used in treatment.

Q307. Answer: B

Explanation: A persecutory delusion involves a fixed false belief that one is being harmed, monitored, or conspired against by others. Individuals firmly believe that outside forces are targeting them despite clear evidence to the contrary. These beliefs are resistant to logical explanation. Persecutory themes are among the most common delusional patterns in psychotic disorders. The conviction may cause severe distress and mistrust of others. Treatment typically involves antipsychotic medication and supportive therapy.

Q308. Answer: A

Explanation: A manic episode involves a period of abnormally elevated or irritable mood with increased energy lasting at least one week. Symptoms include decreased need for sleep, racing thoughts, grandiosity, and impulsive behavior. The severity often causes significant impairment in social or occupational functioning. Hospitalization may be required in severe cases. Mania is a defining feature of bipolar I disorder. Proper management typically includes mood stabilizers or antipsychotic medications.

Q309. Answer: C

Explanation: Obsessive-compulsive disorder is characterized by obsessions and compulsions. Obsessions are intrusive and unwanted thoughts that cause anxiety or distress. Compulsions are repetitive behaviors performed to reduce anxiety triggered by those thoughts. Excessive handwashing related to contamination fears is one of the most common patterns. The behavior temporarily reduces distress but reinforces the cycle of obsession and compulsion. Treatment often includes cognitive behavioral therapy and selective serotonin reuptake inhibitors.

Q310. Answer: C

Explanation: Clozapine is associated with a rare but serious risk of agranulocytosis, a severe reduction in white blood cells. This condition increases susceptibility to life-threatening infections. Because of this risk, routine monitoring of absolute neutrophil count is mandatory. The monitoring program ensures early detection and prevention of complications. Despite this risk, clozapine is highly effective for treatment-resistant schizophrenia. Careful adherence to monitoring guidelines is essential for safe therapy.

Q311. Answer: B

Explanation: Akathisia is a movement disorder characterized by inner restlessness and an inability to remain still. Patients may pace, shift weight frequently, or constantly move their legs. It commonly occurs as an adverse effect of antipsychotic medications. The discomfort can be severe and is often mistaken for anxiety or agitation. Early recognition is important because untreated akathisia may lead to medication non-adherence. Management may involve dose adjustment or medications such as beta-blockers.

Q312. Answer: C

Explanation: Oppositional defiant disorder involves a pattern of angry, defiant, and argumentative behavior toward authority figures. The behavior must persist for at least six months and occur more frequently than typical developmental patterns. Children often deliberately annoy others and refuse to comply with rules. Unlike conduct disorder, the behaviors do not involve serious violations of social norms or aggression toward people or animals. Early intervention can improve outcomes. Behavioral therapy and family interventions are commonly recommended treatments.

Q313. Answer: A

Explanation: Denial is a psychological defense mechanism in which a person refuses to accept reality or facts that cause distress. The individual unconsciously blocks external events from awareness. This response temporarily protects the person from emotional pain or anxiety. However, prolonged denial can interfere with problem solving and adaptation. It is often observed when individuals face serious illness or trauma. Recognition of this defense helps clinicians understand coping patterns.

Q314. Answer: B

Explanation: Acute dystonia is characterized by sudden, sustained muscle contractions leading to abnormal postures. It often affects the neck, jaw, eyes, or back. This reaction typically occurs shortly after initiating or increasing the dose of antipsychotic medication. The symptoms can be distressing and sometimes painful. Prompt treatment with anticholinergic medications such as benztropine is usually effective. Early recognition helps prevent recurrence and improves patient comfort.

Q315. Answer: D

Explanation: Depersonalization involves a sense of detachment from one's own thoughts, feelings, or body. Individuals may feel as though they are observing themselves from outside. Reality testing remains intact, meaning the person recognizes that the experience is unusual. It often occurs during periods of intense stress or trauma. The sensation can be transient or part of a dissociative disorder. Psychological therapies often focus on grounding techniques and stress management.

Q316. Answer: B

Explanation: Serotonin syndrome results from excessive serotonergic activity in the central nervous system. It often occurs when multiple serotonergic medications are combined. Symptoms include agitation, hyperreflexia, tremor, diaphoresis, and autonomic instability. The condition can progress rapidly and become life-threatening if untreated. Management involves discontinuing serotonergic agents and providing supportive care. Early recognition is crucial to prevent complications.

Q317. Answer: A

Explanation: Dopamine plays a major role in the brain's reward and motivation systems. It is involved in reinforcement learning and the experience of pleasure. Dysregulation of dopamine pathways is implicated in several psychiatric conditions. Increased dopaminergic activity is associated with psychotic symptoms such as hallucinations and delusions. Reduced dopamine function may contribute to anhedonia and lack of motivation. Many psychiatric medications target dopamine receptors to restore balance in these pathways.

Q318. Answer: B

Explanation: Antisocial personality disorder involves a pervasive pattern of disregard for the rights of others. Individuals often engage in deceitful, manipulative, or criminal behavior. Lack of empathy and remorse are key characteristics. Symptoms usually begin as conduct problems during childhood or adolescence. The behavior continues into adulthood with repeated violations of social norms. Treatment is challenging and often focuses on behavioral management and risk reduction.

Q319. Answer: A

Explanation: Panic disorder is characterized by recurrent, unexpected panic attacks. These episodes involve sudden surges of intense fear that reach a peak within minutes. Physical symptoms often include palpitations, chest pain, dizziness, and shortness of breath. Individuals may begin to worry about future attacks or change behavior to avoid them. Panic attacks can occur without a clear trigger. Treatment commonly includes cognitive behavioral therapy and pharmacologic interventions.

Q320. Answer: C

Explanation: Negative reinforcement occurs when a behavior is strengthened because it reduces or removes unpleasant feelings. In obsessive-compulsive disorder, compulsive behaviors temporarily relieve anxiety caused by intrusive thoughts. This relief reinforces the behavior and increases the likelihood that it will be repeated. Over time the cycle becomes deeply ingrained. The individual recognizes the behavior as excessive but feels compelled to perform it. Behavioral therapies aim to break this reinforcement pattern through exposure and response prevention.

Q321. Answer: D

Explanation: Negative symptoms involve the absence or reduction of normal emotional and behavioral functions. Examples include flat affect, alogia, avolition, and social withdrawal. These symptoms contrast with positive symptoms such as hallucinations or delusions, which represent excess or distortion of normal functioning. Negative symptoms are often more resistant to treatment. They significantly impair social and occupational functioning. Addressing them often requires a combination of pharmacologic and psychosocial interventions.

Q322. Answer: C

Explanation: Borderline personality disorder is characterized by emotional instability, impulsive behavior, and unstable interpersonal relationships. Individuals often experience intense fears of abandonment. Their self-image may fluctuate dramatically. Mood changes can occur rapidly and are often triggered by interpersonal stress. Self-harm behaviors and chronic feelings of emptiness are also common. Treatment typically focuses on psychotherapy, particularly dialectical behavior therapy.

Q323. Answer: A

Explanation: Antidepressants that inhibit serotonin reuptake increase serotonin levels in the synaptic cleft. However, clinical improvement usually takes several weeks. This delay occurs because therapeutic effects involve neuroadaptive changes within neural circuits. Receptor sensitivity and downstream signaling pathways gradually adjust to the increased neurotransmitter availability. These adaptations enhance emotional regulation and mood stability. The process explains why patients must continue medication despite delayed benefits.

Q324. Answer: B

Explanation: Delusions of reference occur when individuals believe that unrelated events or communications are directed specifically at them. Media broadcasts, conversations, or gestures may be interpreted as personal messages. This misinterpretation reflects a distorted belief about the significance of external events. The conviction remains firm even when evidence contradicts it. Such delusions are commonly associated with schizophrenia and other psychotic disorders. Antipsychotic medications are typically used in treatment.

Q325. Answer: D

Explanation: Social anxiety disorder involves intense fear of situations where an individual may be evaluated by others. The person worries about humiliation, embarrassment, or negative judgment. Social interactions and performance situations often trigger significant distress. As a result, individuals may avoid these situations or endure them with extreme anxiety. The condition can impair occupational and social functioning. Treatment often includes cognitive behavioral therapy and pharmacologic options such as SSRIs.

Q326. Answer: D

Explanation: Tardive dyskinesia is a late-onset movement disorder associated with chronic antipsychotic use. It involves repetitive involuntary movements of the face, lips, tongue, or extremities. The condition results from long-term dopamine receptor blockade leading to receptor supersensitivity. Symptoms may persist even after medication is discontinued. Early detection is important to prevent progression. Treatment may include dose reduction or medications such as VMAT2 inhibitors.

Q327. Answer: C

Explanation: The hypothalamic-pituitary-adrenal axis is the central stress response system. When stress occurs, the hypothalamus releases corticotropin-releasing hormone. This stimulates the pituitary gland to release adrenocorticotropic hormone, which triggers cortisol release from the adrenal glands. Cortisol helps the body respond to stress but prolonged activation can have negative health effects. Chronic elevation may contribute to mood disturbances and fatigue. Dysregulation of this system is associated with several psychiatric disorders.

Q328. Answer: A

Explanation: Dissociative amnesia involves an inability to recall important autobiographical information, usually related to trauma or stress. The memory loss cannot be explained by neurological damage or substance use. Individuals remain conscious and aware but cannot access certain memories. The condition is thought to be a psychological response to overwhelming stress. Recovery may occur spontaneously or with therapeutic intervention. Psychotherapy often focuses on processing trauma and restoring memory integration.

Q329. Answer: A

Explanation: Narcissistic personality disorder is characterized by grandiosity, a strong need for admiration, and limited empathy for others. Individuals often exaggerate achievements and expect recognition without corresponding accomplishments. They may believe they are superior or uniquely talented. Interpersonal relationships can be strained due to arrogance and exploitation. Despite outward confidence, underlying self-esteem may be fragile. Psychotherapy focuses on improving empathy and interpersonal functioning.

Q330. Answer: D

Explanation: Atypical depression is characterized by mood reactivity along with specific vegetative symptoms. Individuals often experience increased appetite, weight gain, hypersomnia, and sensitivity to rejection. These features contrast with melancholic depression, which involves decreased appetite and insomnia. The mood may temporarily improve in response to positive events. This pattern represents a recognized specifier for major depressive episodes. Treatment approaches may include antidepressants and psychotherapy.

Q331. Answer: C

Explanation: Specific phobia involves an intense and irrational fear of a particular object or situation. Exposure to the feared stimulus triggers immediate anxiety or panic. Individuals recognize the fear as excessive but still avoid the situation. Avoidance behavior can interfere with normal functioning. Phobias commonly involve animals, heights, blood, or flying. Exposure-based behavioral therapy is considered the most effective treatment.

Q332. Answer: A

Explanation: Loose associations occur when thoughts shift from one topic to another with little or no logical connection. Speech becomes difficult to follow because ideas are loosely linked or unrelated. This pattern is commonly observed in schizophrenia and other psychotic disorders. The disruption reflects impaired organization of thought processes. Clinicians assess these abnormalities during mental status examinations. Treatment focuses on addressing the underlying psychotic condition.

Q333. Answer: C

Explanation: Illness anxiety disorder involves persistent fear of having or developing a serious illness. Individuals misinterpret normal bodily sensations as signs of severe disease. Medical reassurance and negative test results provide only temporary relief. Unlike somatic symptom disorder, physical symptoms are minimal or absent. The anxiety itself becomes the central problem. Cognitive behavioral therapy is often used to address maladaptive health beliefs and reduce anxiety.

Q334. Answer: D

Explanation: Derealization involves a sense that the external environment is unreal or distorted. Individuals may perceive surroundings as dreamlike, foggy, or visually altered. Despite this sensation, reality testing remains intact. The person understands that the experience is subjective rather than an actual change in the environment. This phenomenon often occurs during severe stress or anxiety. It may also appear in dissociative disorders and panic attacks.

Q335. Answer: B

Explanation: Benzodiazepines enhance the activity of gamma-aminobutyric acid, the main inhibitory neurotransmitter in the brain. They bind to specific receptor sites and increase the frequency of chloride channel opening. This action leads to neuronal hyperpolarization and reduced excitability. The result is a calming effect on the central nervous system. These medications are commonly used for anxiety, insomnia, and acute agitation. However, long-term use carries risks of tolerance and dependence.

Q336. Answer: B

Explanation: Posttraumatic stress disorder develops after exposure to a traumatic event involving threat of death or serious injury. Core symptoms include intrusive memories, nightmares, avoidance behaviors, and heightened arousal. The symptoms persist for more than one month and cause functional impairment. Hypervigilance and exaggerated startle response are common features. Individuals may avoid places or situations that remind them of the trauma. Treatment typically includes trauma-focused psychotherapy and medication when necessary.

Q337. Answer: B

Explanation: Valproate is a mood stabilizer commonly used in the treatment of bipolar disorder. It helps control manic episodes and prevent mood fluctuations. The medication influences several neurotransmitter systems and enhances inhibitory signaling in the brain. By stabilizing neuronal activity, it reduces excessive excitability associated with mania. Valproate is also used in epilepsy and migraine prevention. Monitoring liver function and blood levels is recommended during therapy.

Q338. Answer: C

Explanation: Cognitive symptoms of depression involve negative patterns of thinking and self-evaluation. Individuals often feel worthless, excessively guilty, or pessimistic about the future. These thoughts contribute to low self-esteem and hopelessness. Cognitive distortions can worsen mood and impair decision making. Addressing these patterns is a central component of cognitive behavioral therapy. Improvement in thinking patterns often leads to emotional recovery.

Q339. Answer: B

Explanation: Schizoid personality disorder is characterized by detachment from social relationships and restricted emotional expression. Individuals often prefer solitary activities and show little interest in forming close relationships. They may appear emotionally cold or indifferent to social feedback. Unlike schizophrenia, there are no persistent psychotic symptoms. The pattern typically begins in early adulthood and remains stable over time. Treatment focuses on improving social skills and interpersonal functioning.

Q340. Answer: D

Explanation: Major depressive disorder with seasonal pattern involves recurrent depressive episodes linked to specific times of the year. Symptoms often begin during fall or winter and improve in spring or summer. Reduced sunlight exposure is believed to influence circadian rhythms and neurotransmitter activity. Individuals may experience hypersomnia, increased appetite, and low energy. Light therapy is a commonly recommended treatment. Antidepressant medication may also be helpful in managing symptoms.

Q341. Answer: D

Explanation: Histrionic personality disorder involves excessive emotionality and a strong desire to be the center of attention. Individuals may display dramatic behavior and rapidly shifting emotions. Their speech and interactions often appear theatrical or exaggerated. Relationships may seem superficial because attention-seeking behavior dominates interactions. The need for approval and admiration can influence many aspects of behavior. Psychotherapy is typically the primary treatment approach.

Q342. Answer: B

Explanation: Persistent depressive disorder, previously known as dysthymia, involves a chronic depressed mood lasting at least two years in adults. Symptoms may be less severe than major depressive episodes but are long-lasting. Individuals often report fatigue, low self-esteem, and feelings of hopelessness. The persistent nature of the condition can significantly affect functioning. Periods of normal mood rarely last longer than two months. Treatment may involve psychotherapy and antidepressant medications.

Q343. Answer: C

Explanation: Flight of ideas is characterized by rapid transitions between related topics during speech. Thoughts move quickly, often making it difficult for others to follow the conversation. This pattern is commonly associated with manic episodes in bipolar disorder. Although the ideas may be loosely connected, the speed of thinking and speaking is markedly increased. The symptom reflects heightened cognitive and emotional activity. Treatment focuses on stabilizing the underlying mood disorder.

Q344. Answer: B

Explanation: Behavioral therapy focuses on modifying maladaptive behaviors through structured techniques. Relaxation training, exposure therapy, and reinforcement strategies are common methods used in this approach. Deep breathing and progressive muscle relaxation help reduce physiological arousal associated with anxiety. These techniques teach patients how to manage stress responses effectively.

Over time, repeated practice can decrease anxiety symptoms. Behavioral interventions are frequently combined with cognitive strategies in modern therapy.

Q345. Answer: A

Explanation: Auditory hallucinations involve hearing sounds or voices that are not present in the external environment. They are the most common hallucinations in psychotic disorders. Voices may comment on behavior, converse with each other, or give commands. These experiences are perceived as real by the individual experiencing them. The phenomenon reflects abnormal sensory perception within the brain. Antipsychotic medications are often used to reduce these symptoms.

Q346. Answer: D

Explanation: Obsessive-compulsive personality disorder involves a preoccupation with orderliness, perfectionism, and control. Individuals often become so focused on details and rules that productivity is impaired. The rigidity can interfere with flexibility and efficiency in daily tasks. Unlike obsessive-compulsive disorder, intrusive obsessions and compulsions are not the central features. Instead, the pattern reflects a personality style emphasizing control and precision. Psychotherapy can help patients develop greater flexibility and balance.

Q347. Answer: B

Explanation: Paranoia involves irrational suspicion and mistrust of others. Individuals may believe they are being persecuted, monitored, or harmed by outside forces. These beliefs persist despite clear evidence to the contrary. Paranoid thinking can significantly affect relationships and functioning. It is commonly associated with psychotic disorders but may also appear in personality disorders. Treatment often involves antipsychotic medication and supportive therapy.

Q348. Answer: D

Explanation: Opioids act on receptors that normally respond to endogenous opioid peptides. When opioid use stops suddenly, the body experiences a deficit in these signaling pathways. The nervous system becomes hyperactive due to loss of inhibitory opioid effects. This leads to withdrawal symptoms such as muscle aches, sweating, agitation, and gastrointestinal distress. Although uncomfortable, withdrawal is usually not life-threatening. Treatment may include medications that reduce withdrawal severity.

Q349. Answer: A

Explanation: Dependent personality disorder is characterized by excessive reliance on others for emotional and decision-making support. Individuals often feel incapable of functioning independently. They may have difficulty initiating projects or expressing disagreement due to fear of losing support. This dependence can lead to submissive or clingy behavior in relationships. The pattern typically begins in early adulthood. Psychotherapy aims to increase autonomy and confidence in decision making.

Q350. Answer: A

Explanation: Nihilistic delusions involve beliefs that oneself, parts of the body, or the world no longer exist. Individuals may think they are dead or that their organs are decaying. These beliefs are firmly held despite clear evidence to the contrary. Such delusions are often associated with severe depression or psychotic disorders. The conviction can lead to profound distress and functional impairment. Treatment typically includes antipsychotic medication and management of the underlying condition.

Q351. Answer: C

Explanation: A hypomanic episode involves a distinct period of elevated or irritable mood lasting at least four consecutive days. Symptoms include increased energy, reduced need for sleep, and heightened activity levels. Unlike full mania, hypomania does not cause severe impairment in social or occupational functioning. Hospitalization is typically not required during hypomanic episodes. These episodes are a key feature of bipolar II disorder. Recognition is important because treatment focuses on mood stabilization and prevention of mood cycling.

Q352. Answer: B

Explanation: Trichotillomania is characterized by recurrent pulling out of one's hair, resulting in hair loss. Individuals often feel tension before pulling and relief afterward. The behavior may occur from the scalp, eyebrows, or other body areas. It is classified among obsessive-compulsive and related disorders. Many patients attempt to stop the behavior but struggle to control the urge. Behavioral therapies such as habit reversal training are commonly used in treatment.

Q353. Answer: D

Explanation: Hoarding disorder involves persistent difficulty discarding possessions due to perceived need to save them. This leads to accumulation of items that clutter living areas and impair functioning. Individuals often experience distress at the thought of discarding items. The clutter can create safety hazards and disrupt daily life. Hoarding behavior is distinct from collecting because the items usually lack significant value. Treatment often includes cognitive behavioral therapy focused on decision-making and organization skills.

Q354. Answer: B

Explanation: Bulimia nervosa involves recurrent episodes of binge eating followed by compensatory behaviors. These behaviors may include vomiting, misuse of laxatives, or excessive exercise. Individuals typically feel a loss of control during binge episodes. Unlike anorexia nervosa, body weight often remains within the normal range. The disorder is frequently associated with body image concerns and shame about eating behaviors. Treatment often includes psychotherapy and nutritional counseling.

Q355. Answer: D

Explanation: Agoraphobia involves intense fear of situations where escape might be difficult or help unavailable during panic-like symptoms. Individuals may avoid public transportation, crowds, or being outside alone. The fear often develops after experiencing panic attacks. Avoidance behaviors can become severe enough that patients rarely leave home. The disorder significantly interferes with daily functioning. Treatment commonly includes cognitive behavioral therapy and medication when necessary.

Q356. Answer: D

Explanation: Thought blocking refers to an abrupt interruption in the flow of thought. The person may suddenly stop speaking and appear unable to recall what they were saying. This phenomenon is commonly observed in psychotic disorders such as schizophrenia. It reflects disturbances in the organization or continuity of thought processes. Patients may report that their thoughts were suddenly taken away or disappeared. Recognition of this symptom is important during mental status examination.

Q357. Answer: D

Explanation: Drug-induced parkinsonism results from dopamine blockade caused by antipsychotic medications. Symptoms resemble those seen in Parkinson disease, including rigidity, bradykinesia, and reduced facial expression. Tremor may also occur in some cases. These symptoms usually appear within weeks of starting treatment. The condition results from interference with dopamine pathways involved in motor control. Management may involve dose reduction or medications that restore neurotransmitter balance.

Q358. Answer: A

Explanation: Catatonia is a psychomotor syndrome characterized by abnormal movement or lack of movement. Patients may display immobility, mutism, rigid posture, or resistance to movement. Some individuals maintain unusual postures for prolonged periods. Catatonia can occur in schizophrenia, mood disorders, or medical conditions. Prompt recognition is important because the condition can be life-threatening if untreated. Treatment often includes benzodiazepines or electroconvulsive therapy.

Q359. Answer: B

Explanation: Excoriation disorder involves recurrent skin picking leading to tissue damage. Individuals often attempt to stop but find it difficult to control the behavior. The behavior may occur in response to stress or perceived skin imperfections. It is categorized among obsessive-compulsive and related disorders. The condition can lead to infections and scarring. Behavioral therapy is commonly used to address the repetitive behavior.

Q360. Answer: C

Explanation: Thought broadcasting is a psychotic symptom in which individuals believe their thoughts are accessible to others. They may feel that their thoughts are transmitted or publicly known. This belief reflects a disturbance in the perception of personal boundaries between self and others. It is commonly associated with schizophrenia and other psychotic disorders. The experience often leads to anxiety and social withdrawal. Treatment generally includes antipsychotic medications and supportive therapy.

Q361. Answer: A

Explanation: Anhedonia refers to the inability to experience pleasure from activities that were previously enjoyable. It is one of the core symptoms of major depressive disorder. Individuals may lose interest in hobbies, social interactions, or other rewarding experiences. This symptom reflects dysfunction in the brain's reward pathways. It often contributes to social withdrawal and reduced motivation. Effective treatment of depression often leads to gradual improvement in the ability to feel pleasure.

Q362. Answer: B

Explanation: Binge eating disorder involves recurrent episodes of consuming unusually large amounts of food in a short period. Individuals often feel a loss of control during these episodes. Unlike bulimia nervosa, there are no regular compensatory behaviors such as vomiting or excessive exercise. Episodes are typically accompanied by feelings of guilt or distress. The condition is associated with obesity and metabolic complications. Treatment includes psychotherapy and nutritional counseling.

Q363. Answer: C

Explanation: Avoidant personality disorder involves intense feelings of inadequacy and hypersensitivity to negative evaluation. Individuals strongly desire relationships but avoid social interactions due to fear of rejection or criticism. The pattern leads to social isolation and limited interpersonal connections. Low self-esteem is a common feature. The condition often begins in early adulthood and persists over time. Psychotherapy focusing on confidence and social skills can be beneficial.

Q364. Answer: C

Explanation: Intermittent explosive disorder is characterized by recurrent episodes of impulsive aggression. The outbursts are disproportionate to the triggering event. Episodes may involve verbal aggression, property destruction, or physical assault. Individuals often feel remorse or embarrassment afterward. The behavior is not premeditated and occurs suddenly. Treatment typically includes psychotherapy and sometimes medication to reduce impulsivity.

Q365. Answer: B

Explanation: Neologisms are newly invented words that have meaning only to the person using them. They are often observed in schizophrenia and other psychotic disorders. The creation of these words reflects disturbances in thought and language organization. Listeners usually cannot understand the meaning because the words are not part of standard language. This symptom is typically identified during clinical interviews. Treatment focuses on managing the underlying psychotic disorder.

Q366. Answer: C

Explanation: Thought insertion involves the belief that external forces are placing thoughts into one's mind. Individuals feel that the thoughts do not originate from themselves. This symptom reflects a breakdown in the sense of ownership over thoughts. It is commonly associated with schizophrenia and related psychotic disorders. The experience can cause significant distress and confusion. Treatment generally involves antipsychotic medication and supportive care.

Q367. Answer: C

Explanation: Body dysmorphic disorder involves excessive concern with perceived defects in physical appearance. The flaws are either minor or not observable to others. Individuals may spend excessive time checking mirrors or seeking reassurance. The preoccupation can cause significant distress and impair functioning. Many patients seek cosmetic procedures in an attempt to correct the perceived flaw. Cognitive behavioral therapy and certain medications are often used in treatment.

Q368. Answer: D

Explanation: Borderline personality disorder involves instability in emotions, behavior, and relationships. Individuals frequently report chronic feelings of emptiness. Impulsive behaviors such as substance use or reckless spending are common. Emotional responses may shift rapidly and intensely. Fear of abandonment often contributes to relationship difficulties. Psychotherapy, especially dialectical behavior therapy, is considered the most effective treatment approach.

Q369. Answer: A

Explanation: Delusions of reference occur when individuals believe that neutral events have personal significance directed toward them. Everyday occurrences such as conversations, gestures, or media broadcasts may be interpreted as hidden messages. These beliefs persist despite evidence showing that the events are unrelated to the individual. This symptom is frequently seen in psychotic disorders. It can lead to suspiciousness and social withdrawal. Treatment focuses on managing the underlying psychosis.

Q370. Answer: A

Explanation: Major depressive disorder with psychotic features involves the presence of delusions or hallucinations during a depressive episode. The psychotic content often reflects themes of guilt, worthlessness, or punishment. These symptoms indicate a more severe form of depression. The condition requires prompt treatment due to increased risk of suicide and functional impairment. Management typically includes antidepressant and antipsychotic medications or electroconvulsive therapy in severe cases.

Q371. Answer: B

Explanation: Echolalia refers to the automatic repetition of another person's spoken words. It is often observed in certain psychiatric and neurological conditions. Individuals may echo phrases immediately or after a delay. The behavior reflects disturbances in language processing or social communication. Echolalia is sometimes seen in catatonia, autism spectrum disorder, or schizophrenia. Recognition of the symptom helps guide clinical evaluation.

Q372. Answer: D

Explanation: Paranoid personality disorder involves pervasive distrust and suspicion of others. Individuals often interpret others' actions as deliberately threatening or harmful. They may hold grudges and remain reluctant to confide in others. The mistrust persists even without evidence of wrongdoing. Relationships are often strained because of the constant suspicion. Psychotherapy can help address maladaptive thinking patterns and interpersonal difficulties.

Q373. Answer: A

Explanation: Histrionic personality disorder is marked by excessive emotional expression and attention-seeking behavior. Individuals may appear theatrical or dramatic in social interactions. Their emotions often shift rapidly and may seem exaggerated. They frequently seek reassurance and approval from others. Relationships may appear intense but superficial. Psychotherapy is the primary treatment method used to address these patterns.

Q374. Answer: B

Explanation: Grandiose delusions involve exaggerated beliefs about one's importance, power, or identity. Individuals may believe they possess special talents or abilities beyond reality. These beliefs remain fixed despite evidence contradicting them. Grandiosity may occur in manic episodes or psychotic disorders. The conviction often leads to unrealistic plans or risky decisions. Treatment focuses on stabilizing mood and addressing psychotic symptoms.

Q375. Answer: A

Explanation: Oculogyric crisis is a form of acute dystonia involving involuntary upward deviation of the eyes. It is commonly associated with antipsychotic medications. The reaction occurs due to dopamine receptor blockade affecting motor control pathways. Symptoms can be distressing but are usually reversible with treatment. Anticholinergic medications are often used to relieve the muscle spasms. Early recognition helps prevent prolonged discomfort.

Q376. Answer: D

Explanation: Adjustment disorder occurs when emotional or behavioral symptoms develop in response to a specific stressor. The distress is greater than expected and interferes with normal functioning. Symptoms begin within three months of the stressor. However, the individual does not meet criteria for another psychiatric disorder. Once the stressor resolves, symptoms typically improve. Psychotherapy is often helpful in developing coping strategies.

Q377. Answer: B

Explanation: Antisocial personality disorder involves a consistent pattern of disregard for the rights of others. Individuals often engage in deceitful or manipulative behavior. Lack of empathy and remorse are key characteristics. Many individuals have a history of conduct problems during adolescence. The behavior frequently leads to legal or interpersonal difficulties. Treatment focuses on behavioral management and addressing risk behaviors.

Q378. Answer: A

Explanation: Delirium is an acute disturbance in attention and awareness. Symptoms develop rapidly and fluctuate throughout the day. Individuals may experience confusion, disorientation, and altered consciousness. The condition often results from medical illness, infection, or medication effects. Unlike dementia, delirium develops suddenly and is often reversible. Prompt identification and treatment of the underlying cause are essential.

Q379. Answer: C

Explanation: Command hallucinations involve voices instructing the individual to perform specific actions. These auditory experiences can be particularly concerning when they encourage harmful behaviors. They are most commonly associated with psychotic disorders. Patients may feel compelled to obey the voices because they perceive them as powerful or authoritative. Assessment of safety risk is essential when this symptom occurs. Treatment includes antipsychotic medication and close monitoring.

Q380. Answer: B

Explanation: Perseveration refers to the persistent repetition of a particular response or topic. The individual continues to focus on the same idea even when the conversation has moved on. This symptom can occur in several psychiatric and neurological conditions. It reflects difficulty shifting attention or cognitive flexibility. Perseveration may interfere with effective communication. Identifying the pattern helps clinicians evaluate cognitive and thought processes.

Q381. Answer: A

Explanation: A panic attack is a sudden surge of intense fear or discomfort that reaches a peak within minutes. Physical symptoms often include palpitations, sweating, trembling, and shortness of breath. Individuals may also feel a sense of impending doom or loss of control. These episodes can occur unexpectedly or in response to specific triggers. Panic attacks are common in several anxiety disorders. Treatment may involve psychotherapy and medications that regulate anxiety symptoms.

Q382. Answer: A

Explanation: Cognitive distortions involve irrational or exaggerated patterns of thinking. In depression, individuals may interpret minor events as evidence of personal failure or guilt. These distorted beliefs reinforce negative self-perception and hopelessness. They often contribute to the persistence of depressive symptoms. Cognitive behavioral therapy specifically targets these thinking patterns. By challenging distorted beliefs, patients can develop healthier perspectives and improve mood.

Q383. Answer: A

Explanation: Schizoid personality disorder is characterized by detachment from social relationships. Individuals often prefer solitary activities and show little desire for close friendships. Emotional expression may appear restricted or flat. Unlike avoidant personality disorder, these individuals typically do not feel distressed about isolation. The pattern usually begins in early adulthood and remains consistent over time. Treatment may focus on improving social functioning when desired by the patient.

Q384. Answer: A

Explanation: Waxy flexibility is a feature of catatonia in which a person maintains positions placed by another individual. The limbs may remain in unusual postures for extended periods. Resistance to movement is minimal, and the body appears flexible like soft wax. This symptom reflects severe psychomotor disturbance. It is most often seen in catatonic states associated with psychiatric disorders. Treatment frequently involves benzodiazepines or electroconvulsive therapy.

Q385. Answer: A

Explanation: Somatic delusions involve false beliefs about bodily functions or sensations. Individuals may believe that their body is diseased, deformed, or emitting unpleasant odors. These beliefs persist despite medical evidence showing no abnormality. Somatic delusions can occur in psychotic disorders or severe mood disorders. The conviction often causes distress and social avoidance. Treatment generally includes antipsychotic medication and supportive therapy.

Q386. Answer: C

Explanation: Serotonin syndrome occurs when excessive serotonergic activity develops in the central nervous system. It is commonly triggered by combining medications that increase serotonin levels. Symptoms include agitation, tremor, sweating, and elevated body temperature. Neuromuscular abnormalities such as hyperreflexia are also common. The condition can progress rapidly and become life-threatening. Immediate discontinuation of serotonergic agents and supportive treatment are required.

Q387. Answer: D

Explanation: Borderline personality disorder often involves unstable interpersonal relationships. Individuals may alternate between idealizing and devaluing others. This pattern reflects difficulty maintaining stable perceptions of relationships. Fear of abandonment frequently contributes to these rapid shifts. Emotional intensity and impulsivity are also common features. Psychotherapy focusing on emotional regulation is the main treatment approach.

Q388. Answer: B

Explanation: Negative reinforcement strengthens behavior because it removes an unpleasant emotional state. In obsessive-compulsive disorder, compulsive actions reduce anxiety triggered by intrusive thoughts. The temporary relief reinforces the behavior and makes it more likely to occur again. Over time, this cycle strengthens the compulsion. The individual recognizes the behavior as excessive but feels compelled to perform it. Behavioral therapy focuses on breaking this cycle through exposure and response prevention.

Q389. Answer: C

Explanation: Bipolar II disorder involves at least one major depressive episode and one hypomanic episode. Unlike bipolar I disorder, there are no full manic episodes. Hypomania produces noticeable changes in mood and energy but does not cause severe impairment. Depressive episodes are often the most disabling component of the disorder. Accurate diagnosis is important because treatment focuses on mood stabilization. Management often includes mood stabilizers and psychotherapy.

Q390. Answer: D

Explanation: Catatonia is a psychomotor syndrome involving abnormal movement or behavior. Patients may exhibit immobility, mutism, or resistance to movement. The condition can occur in psychiatric disorders such as schizophrenia or mood disorders. It may also arise from medical conditions. Recognition is critical because untreated catatonia can lead to complications such as dehydration or malnutrition. Benzodiazepines and electroconvulsive therapy are common treatments.

Q391. Answer: B

Explanation: Dependent personality disorder is characterized by excessive reliance on others for emotional support and decision-making. Individuals fear separation and may feel helpless when alone. They often seek reassurance and approval from others. Difficulty making independent decisions is a common feature. This dependency can lead to submissive behavior in relationships. Psychotherapy aims to strengthen self-confidence and independence.

Q392. Answer: A

Explanation: Palilalia refers to the repetition of one's own words or phrases. The repetitions may occur rapidly and multiple times. This speech pattern can occur in certain neurological and psychiatric conditions. It reflects disturbances in speech regulation and cognitive control. Palilalia differs from echolalia, where a person repeats another individual's words. Identifying the pattern helps clinicians assess language abnormalities.

Q393. Answer: B

Explanation: Major depressive disorder involves persistent low mood or loss of interest in activities for at least two weeks. Additional symptoms often include fatigue, sleep disturbance, and feelings of hopelessness. The condition significantly interferes with daily functioning. Biological, psychological, and social factors contribute to its development. Effective treatments include antidepressant medications and psychotherapy. Early intervention improves outcomes and reduces the risk of recurrence.

Q394. Answer: A

Explanation: Persecutory delusions involve false beliefs that others intend to harm, harass, or conspire against the individual. These beliefs are held firmly despite contradictory evidence. The person may feel constantly threatened or monitored. Persecutory themes are among the most common types of delusions in psychotic disorders. The beliefs often lead to suspiciousness and social withdrawal. Treatment typically involves antipsychotic medication and supportive therapy.

Q395. Answer: A

Explanation: Tactile hallucinations involve sensations of touch without an external stimulus. Individuals may feel crawling, burning, or tingling sensations on the skin. The experience can be distressing and may lead to scratching or attempts to remove the perceived source. Tactile hallucinations may occur in certain psychiatric or substance-related conditions. Careful evaluation is required to determine the underlying cause. Treatment focuses on addressing the primary disorder responsible for the symptom.

Q396. Answer: B

Explanation: Narcissistic personality disorder is characterized by grandiosity and a strong need for admiration. Individuals often exaggerate accomplishments and believe they deserve special treatment. They may show limited empathy for others. Relationships can become strained due to arrogance or entitlement. Despite apparent confidence, self-esteem may be fragile. Psychotherapy can help improve empathy and interpersonal functioning.

Q397. Answer: C

Explanation: Obsessive-compulsive disorder involves intrusive thoughts and repetitive behaviors performed to reduce anxiety. Some individuals experience obsessions related to symmetry or order. Compulsive actions such as arranging or aligning objects temporarily relieve distress. However, the relief reinforces the behavior and perpetuates the cycle. The condition can significantly interfere with daily functioning. Cognitive behavioral therapy and medication are common treatment options.

Q398. Answer: D

Explanation: Dissociative fugue involves sudden travel away from one's usual environment accompanied by memory loss for personal identity. The individual may appear normal to others but cannot recall their past. The condition is often triggered by severe stress or trauma. During the episode, the person may assume a new identity or role. Recovery typically involves gradual return of memory. Psychotherapy focuses on processing the underlying stressor and restoring identity continuity.

Q399. Answer: D

Explanation: Thought withdrawal is a psychotic symptom in which individuals believe that their thoughts are being taken away by outside forces. The experience creates a sense that thoughts disappear suddenly or are stolen. It reflects a disturbance in the perception of ownership of mental processes. This symptom is commonly associated with schizophrenia and related disorders. The belief is firmly held despite lack of evidence. Antipsychotic medications are typically used in treatment.

Q400. Answer: C

Explanation: Antidepressant medications often increase neurotransmitter availability shortly after administration. However, clinical improvement usually requires several weeks. The delay occurs because long-term changes in receptor sensitivity and intracellular signaling must develop. These neuroadaptive processes modify communication between brain regions involved in mood regulation. Over time, these changes restore more balanced emotional processing. This gradual adjustment explains why patients are advised to continue medication even when early effects are not immediately noticeable.

Question (401-500)

Q401. A 25-year-old patient presents with decreased need for sleep, excessive goal-directed activity, pressured speech, and impulsive spending for the past 6 days. The patient reports feeling unusually confident and energetic but denies hallucinations or delusions. Which diagnosis is most consistent with these findings?

(A) Cyclothymic disorder
(B) Bipolar I disorder
(C) Bipolar II disorder
(D) Persistent depressive disorder

Q402. A patient treated with a first-generation antipsychotic develops sustained neck muscle contractions and painful twisting of the head shortly after receiving the medication. What condition is the patient most likely experiencing?

(A) Neuroleptic malignant syndrome
(B) Tardive dyskinesia
(C) Acute dystonia
(D) Akathisia

Q403. A clinician evaluating a patient with depressive symptoms administers the PHQ-9 screening tool. What is the primary purpose of this instrument?

(A) Diagnose bipolar disorder
(B) Identify personality disorders
(C) Screen and monitor depression severity
(D) Measure cognitive impairment

Q404. A patient experiencing alcohol withdrawal demonstrates tremors, diaphoresis, tachycardia, and agitation. Which clinical scale is most appropriate for assessing the severity of this condition?

(A) PHQ-9
(B) GAD-7
(C) CIWA-Ar
(D) MMSE

Q405. During a mental status examination, a patient states that the television news anchor is sending them secret personal messages through the broadcast. This symptom represents which type of psychopathology?

(A) Circumstantial speech
(B) Delusion of reference
(C) Thought blocking
(D) Illusion

Q406. A patient receiving lithium therapy presents with nausea, tremor, confusion, and unsteady gait. What is the most appropriate initial action?

(A) Administer benzodiazepines
(B) Initiate antidepressant therapy
(C) Continue medication and monitor symptoms
(D) Obtain serum lithium level immediately

Q407. A clinician explains to a patient that therapy will focus on identifying negative thought patterns and replacing them with more adaptive beliefs. Which psychotherapy approach is being described?

(A) Gestalt therapy
(B) Cognitive behavioral therapy
(C) Psychoanalysis
(D) Existential therapy

Q408. A patient reports feeling restless and unable to sit still after starting a new antipsychotic medication. The patient constantly paces and describes an inner sense of agitation. Which adverse effect is most likely occurring?
(A) Akathisia
(B) Parkinsonism
(C) Dystonia
(D) Serotonin syndrome
Q409. A patient expresses a desire to end their life and reports having access to a firearm at home. What is the clinician's priority intervention?
(A) Prescribe antidepressant medication
(B) Conduct immediate suicide risk assessment and safety planning
(C) Schedule follow-up appointment
(D) Begin psychotherapy session
Q410. A patient with generalized anxiety disorder reports persistent worry about multiple life events for more than six months accompanied by fatigue, irritability, and sleep disturbance. Which neurotransmitter imbalance is most strongly associated with this condition?
(A) Hypertensive crisis
(B) Serotonin syndrome
(C) Neuroleptic malignant syndrome
(D) Acute dystonia
Q411. A patient reports hearing voices that comment on their behavior even when no one else is present. What type of perceptual disturbance is this?
(A) Illusion
(B) Delusion
(C) Auditory hallucination
(D) Confabulation
Q412. During a mental status examination, a patient abruptly stops speaking in the middle of a sentence and appears unable to recall what they were saying. Which term best describes this finding?
(A) Tangentiality
(B) Flight of ideas
(C) Thought blocking
(D) Perseveration
Q413. A clinician suspects major depressive disorder in a patient who reports persistent sadness, diminished interest in activities, fatigue, and poor concentration for two months. What diagnostic requirement must also be present?
(A) Significant distress or impairment in functioning
(B) Presence of psychotic features
(C) At least one manic episode
(D) Symptoms lasting at least two years
Q414. A patient treated with an antipsychotic develops muscle rigidity, hyperthermia, altered consciousness, and autonomic instability. What condition should the clinician suspect?
(A) Acute akathisia
(B) Malignant hyperthermia
(C) Neuroleptic malignant syndrome
(D) Serotonin syndrome
Q415. A patient describes experiencing persistent feelings of emptiness, unstable relationships, impulsive behavior, and intense fear of abandonment. Which personality disorder is most consistent with these features?

(A) Avoidant personality disorder
(B) Schizoid personality disorder
(C) Borderline personality disorder
(D) Narcissistic personality disorder

Q416. A patient undergoing opioid withdrawal experiences yawning, rhinorrhea, muscle aches, and restlessness. Which clinical scale is most commonly used to assess withdrawal severity?
(A) COWS
(B) GAD-7
(C) PHQ-9
(D) HAM-D

Q417. A patient reports hearing voices commenting on their actions when no one else is present. What type of hallucination is being described?
(A) Auditory hallucination
(B) Visual hallucination
(C) Olfactory hallucination
(D) Tactile hallucination

Q418. A patient receiving selective serotonin reuptake inhibitor therapy develops agitation, tremor, hyperreflexia, and fever after starting another serotonergic medication. What condition should be suspected?
(A) Serotonin syndrome
(B) Hypertensive crisis
(C) Lithium toxicity
(D) Anticholinergic toxicity

Q419. During an interview, a patient provides excessive unnecessary detail but eventually returns to the original question. Which speech pattern does this represent?
(A) Word salad
(B) Neologism
(C) Circumstantiality
(D) Tangentiality

Q420. A patient reports persistent low mood for more than two years with poor appetite, low energy, and low self-esteem but no history of mania. Which diagnosis is most likely?
(A) Bipolar II disorder
(B) Cyclothymic disorder
(C) Persistent depressive disorder
(D) Acute stress disorder

Q421. A patient experiencing severe anxiety before public speaking practices controlled breathing and progressive muscle relaxation. What therapeutic approach does this technique represent?
(A) Interpersonal therapy
(B) Behavioral therapy
(C) Family systems therapy
(D) Psychoanalytic therapy

Q422. A clinician evaluates whether a patient can understand information about treatment, appreciate consequences, reason about options, and communicate a choice. What is being assessed?
(A) Cognitive intelligence
(B) Personality functioning
(C) Insight level
(D) Decision-making capacity

Q423. A patient treated with haloperidol develops bradykinesia, rigidity, and resting tremor resembling Parkinson disease. Which adverse effect is occurring?
(A) Tardive dyskinesia
(B) Akathisia
(C) Drug-induced parkinsonism
(D) Acute dystonia
Q424. A therapist encourages a patient to explore unconscious conflicts originating in childhood experiences. Which therapeutic model is being used?
(A) Behavioral therapy
(B) Solution-focused therapy
(C) Psychoanalytic therapy
(D) Cognitive therapy
Q425. A patient with panic disorder experiences sudden episodes of intense fear accompanied by palpitations, chest discomfort, and shortness of breath. What neurotransmitter system is primarily implicated?
(A) Acetylcholine
(B) Histamine
(C) Serotonin and norepinephrine
(D) Glycine
Q426. A clinician warns a patient that abruptly stopping benzodiazepines after prolonged use may result in rebound anxiety, tremors, and seizures. What concept explains this phenomenon?
(A) Drug allergy
(B) Pharmacokinetic tolerance
(C) Placebo response
(D) Physiological dependence
Q427. A patient reports smelling burning rubber despite no identifiable odor source. What type of hallucination is this?
(A) Auditory hallucination
(B) Olfactory hallucination
(C) Gustatory hallucination
(D) Tactile hallucination
Q428. A patient repeatedly checks that the door is locked dozens of times each night despite knowing it is secure. Which disorder most closely matches this behavior?
(A) Generalized anxiety disorder
(B) Obsessive-compulsive disorder
(C) Somatic symptom disorder
(D) Social anxiety disorder
Q429. A patient states that external forces are controlling their thoughts and inserting ideas into their mind. Which symptom is present?
(A) Thought insertion
(B) Confabulation
(C) Derealization
(D) Depersonalization
Q430. A patient presents with confusion, disorientation, fluctuating consciousness, and impaired attention developing over several hours. What condition is most likely?
(A) Dementia
(B) Delirium
(C) Major depressive disorder

(D) Personality disorder

Q431. A patient diagnosed with schizophrenia demonstrates diminished emotional expression, limited speech, and lack of motivation. These findings represent which category of symptoms?

(A) Negative symptoms
(B) Affective symptoms
(C) Positive symptoms
(D) Cognitive symptoms

Q432. A patient with major depressive disorder reports waking up several hours earlier than usual and being unable to return to sleep. What sleep disturbance is this?

(A) Circadian rhythm disorder
(B) Terminal insomnia
(C) Sleep paralysis
(D) Sleep apnea

Q433. A patient suddenly develops severe confusion, hallucinations, and autonomic instability after abrupt cessation of heavy alcohol use. What condition is most likely occurring?

(A) Alcohol intoxication
(B) Delirium tremens
(C) Substance-induced psychosis
(D) Acute stress disorder

Q434. A patient describes feeling detached from their body and observing themselves as if from outside. Which phenomenon is being experienced?

(A) Confabulation
(B) Depersonalization
(C) Dissociation
(D) Derealization

Q435. A clinician instructs a patient with social anxiety disorder to gradually confront feared social situations while practicing coping strategies. What therapy technique is this?

(A) Free association
(B) Exposure therapy
(C) Dream analysis
(D) Hypnosis

Q436. A patient frequently shifts conversation topics rapidly with minimal logical connection between ideas during a manic episode. What speech pattern is this?

(A) Thought blocking
(B) Neologism
(C) Tangentiality
(D) Flight of ideas

Q437. A patient taking clozapine requires routine blood monitoring primarily to detect which serious adverse effect?

(A) Hypertension
(B) Hyperthyroidism
(C) Renal failure
(D) Agranulocytosis

Q438. A patient complains of severe restlessness and an inability to remain seated shortly after starting antipsychotic therapy. What medication class is often used to manage this condition?

(A) Antiviral agents
(B) Antibiotics
(C) Antihistamines

(D) Beta blockers

Q439. A patient believes that strangers on the street are secretly plotting against them without evidence. Which type of delusion is present?

(A) Persecutory delusion
(B) Somatic delusion
(C) Grandiose delusion
(D) Nihilistic delusion

Q440. A patient repeatedly imitates the movements and gestures of the examiner during a psychiatric assessment. What behavior is this called?

(A) Echopraxia
(B) Echolalia
(C) Catatonia
(D) Automatism

Q441. A patient reports persistent fear of being embarrassed in social situations and avoids interacting with unfamiliar people. Which disorder is most consistent with this presentation?

(A) Generalized anxiety disorder
(B) Panic disorder
(C) Social anxiety disorder
(D) Illness anxiety disorder

Q442. A patient with dementia frequently fabricates stories to fill gaps in memory without the intention to deceive. What is this phenomenon called?

(A) Delusion
(B) Confabulation
(C) Illusion
(D) Hallucination

Q443. A patient taking an SSRI complains of decreased libido and difficulty achieving orgasm. What is the most likely explanation?

(A) Hormonal imbalance
(B) Nutritional deficiency
(C) Medication side effect
(D) Neurologic disorder

Q444. A patient describes persistent worry about health despite normal medical evaluations and reassurance from physicians. Which disorder is most consistent with this pattern?

(A) Factitious disorder
(B) Illness anxiety disorder
(C) Conversion disorder
(D) Somatic symptom disorder

Q445. A patient with schizophrenia begins displaying repetitive lip smacking, tongue protrusion, and involuntary facial movements after long-term antipsychotic therapy. What condition is most likely present?

(A) Drug-induced parkinsonism
(B) Tardive dyskinesia
(C) Akathisia
(D) Acute dystonia

Q446. A patient becomes extremely anxious when separated from family members and fears that harm will come to them. Which disorder most closely matches this presentation?

(A) Separation anxiety disorder
(B) Adjustment disorder

(C) Panic disorder
(D) Specific phobia

Q447. A patient reports intense sadness, loss of pleasure, fatigue, and impaired concentration for several weeks following the death of a spouse. Which condition is most appropriate to consider?
(A) Neurocognitive disorder
(B) Normal grief reaction
(C) Psychotic disorder
(D) Bipolar disorder

Q448. A therapist helps a patient identify personal strengths and build resilience in coping with life challenges. Which therapeutic approach emphasizes this perspective?
(A) Hypnotherapy
(B) Behavioral modification
(C) Strength-based therapy
(D) Psychoanalysis

Q449. A patient reports seeing shadows moving in the room but later realizes they were caused by shifting light patterns. What type of perceptual disturbance occurred?
(A) Confabulation
(B) Delusion
(C) Illusion
(D) Hallucination

Q450. A patient undergoing therapy learns techniques to tolerate distress and regulate intense emotions. Which psychotherapy model emphasizes these skills?
(A) Existential therapy
(B) Gestalt therapy
(C) Dialectical behavior therapy
(D) Psychoanalytic therapy

Q451. A patient complains of persistent fatigue, increased appetite, hypersomnia, and sensitivity to rejection during depressive episodes. Which subtype of depression is suggested?
(A) Atypical features
(B) Seasonal pattern
(C) Psychotic features
(D) Melancholic features

Q452. A patient with bipolar disorder reports alternating periods of elevated mood and depressive episodes over several years. Which neurotransmitter systems are most closely involved?
(A) Dopamine, serotonin, and norepinephrine
(B) Glycine and glutamate only
(C) Endorphins exclusively
(D) Histamine and acetylcholine

Q453. A patient repeatedly pulls out their hair resulting in noticeable hair loss and significant distress. Which disorder is most consistent with this behavior?
(A) Body dysmorphic disorder
(B) Trichotillomania
(C) Adjustment disorder
(D) Hoarding disorder

Q454. A patient believes their organs are rotting inside their body despite medical evidence to the contrary. Which type of delusion is this?
(A) Grandiose delusion
(B) Referential delusion

(C) Somatic delusion
(D) Erotomanic delusion

Q455. A patient demonstrates difficulty planning, organizing, and completing complex tasks following a traumatic brain injury. Which cognitive function is most affected?
(A) Motor coordination
(B) Sensory perception
(C) Executive functioning
(D) Visual acuity

Q456. A therapist encourages a patient to focus on present awareness and nonjudgmental acceptance of thoughts and feelings. Which technique is being applied?
(A) Projective testing
(B) Dream interpretation
(C) Mindfulness training
(D) Classical conditioning

Q457. A patient reports recurrent nightmares and intrusive memories several months after experiencing a serious car accident. Which disorder should be considered?
(A) Adjustment disorder
(B) Panic disorder
(C) Acute stress disorder
(D) Posttraumatic stress disorder

Q458. A patient complains of persistent difficulty falling asleep due to racing thoughts and anxiety. Which sleep disorder is most consistent with this description?
(A) Insomnia disorder
(B) Parasomnia
(C) Narcolepsy
(D) Sleep apnea

Q459. A patient frequently accumulates large amounts of unnecessary items and becomes distressed when asked to discard them. Which disorder best describes this behavior?
(A) Body dysmorphic disorder
(B) Illness anxiety disorder
(C) Obsessive-compulsive disorder
(D) Hoarding disorder

Q460. A clinician considers cultural beliefs and values when developing a treatment plan for a patient. What principle is being applied?
(A) Clinical detachment
(B) Cultural competence
(C) Diagnostic overshadowing
(D) Therapeutic neutrality

Q461. A patient taking lithium therapy reports excessive thirst, frequent urination, and mild tremor. Which laboratory test is most important to monitor regularly during treatment?
(A) Serum lithium concentration
(B) Hemoglobin level
(C) Platelet count
(D) Serum calcium level

Q462. A patient with schizophrenia suddenly becomes immobile, maintains a rigid posture for long periods, and does not respond to verbal instructions. Which condition best explains these symptoms?
(A) Delirium
(B) Somatization

(C) Akathisia
(D) Catatonia

Q463. A patient complains of excessive daytime sleepiness and sudden episodes of muscle weakness triggered by laughter. Which disorder is most consistent with these symptoms?
(A) Restless legs syndrome
(B) Insomnia disorder
(C) Sleep apnea
(D) Narcolepsy

Q464. A patient persistently believes they possess extraordinary powers and a special mission to save humanity. What type of delusion is present?
(A) Persecutory delusion
(B) Grandiose delusion
(C) Referential delusion
(D) Somatic delusion

Q465. A patient describes repeatedly washing their hands for hours due to fears of contamination. Which psychological mechanism best explains this behavior?
(A) Delusion
(B) Compulsion
(C) Hallucination
(D) Dissociation

Q466. A patient experiencing panic attacks begins avoiding crowded places because they fear escape would be difficult during an episode. Which condition is suggested?
(A) Separation anxiety disorder
(B) Social anxiety disorder
(C) Agoraphobia
(D) Specific phobia

Q467. A patient demonstrates rapid mood swings, intense anger, and impulsive behavior in relationships. Which therapy approach is most effective for managing these symptoms?
(A) Gestalt therapy
(B) Supportive counseling
(C) Psychoanalytic therapy
(D) Dialectical behavior therapy

Q468. A patient with major depressive disorder reports feeling worse in the morning but gradually improves throughout the day. Which depressive feature does this describe?
(A) Diurnal mood variation
(B) Psychomotor retardation
(C) Seasonal pattern
(D) Circadian rhythm disorder

Q469. A patient experiencing a psychotic episode begins creating new words that have meaning only to them. What speech disturbance is this called?
(A) Echolalia
(B) Circumstantiality
(C) Perseveration
(D) Neologism

Q470. A patient frequently repeats the same phrase or answer regardless of the question asked. Which speech pattern is being demonstrated?
(A) Perseveration
(B) Clang association

(C) Thought blocking
(D) Tangentiality

Q471. A patient complains of persistent sadness, loss of appetite, insomnia, and lack of interest in activities for three weeks. Which diagnosis should be considered first?
(A) Major depressive disorder
(B) Bipolar disorder
(C) Cyclothymic disorder
(D) Schizoaffective disorder

Q472. A patient who experienced severe trauma avoids reminders of the event and feels emotionally numb. Which psychological response does this represent?
(A) Dissociation
(B) Delusion
(C) Hallucination
(D) Catatonia

Q473. A clinician evaluates the ability of a patient to recall three objects after five minutes during a mental status examination. Which cognitive domain is being tested?
(A) Memory
(B) Insight
(C) Language
(D) Judgment

Q474. A patient reports feeling detached from their surroundings, describing the environment as unreal or dreamlike. What phenomenon is this?
(A) Derealization
(B) Illusion
(C) Confabulation
(D) Depersonalization

Q475. A patient diagnosed with bipolar disorder begins taking a medication that stabilizes mood and reduces manic episodes. Which class of medication is most likely prescribed?
(A) Antiviral
(B) Mood stabilizer
(C) Antibiotic
(D) Antihistamine

Q476. A patient repeatedly checks appliances before leaving home because they fear causing a fire. What psychological feature is driving this behavior?
(A) Obsession
(B) Delusion
(C) Phobia
(D) Hallucination

Q477. A patient with dementia becomes disoriented at night and attempts to leave the house believing it is daytime. Which symptom is this called?
(A) Catatonia
(B) Hypomania
(C) Sundowning
(D) Echolalia

Q478. A patient complains of persistent worry about numerous daily events for more than six months. Which disorder is most consistent with this presentation?
(A) Panic disorder
(B) Specific phobia

(C) Generalized anxiety disorder
(D) Social anxiety disorder

Q479. A patient with schizophrenia shows significant impairment in attention, memory, and problem solving. These deficits represent which type of symptoms?
(A) Affective symptoms
(B) Negative symptoms
(C) Cognitive symptoms
(D) Positive symptoms

Q480. A patient experiences persistent sadness during winter months that improves during spring and summer. Which disorder pattern is suggested?
(A) Seasonal pattern depression
(B) Cyclothymic disorder
(C) Persistent depressive disorder
(D) Bipolar disorder

Q481. A therapist encourages a patient to examine how interpersonal relationships influence emotional experiences. Which therapy model is being applied?
(A) Psychoanalysis
(B) Gestalt therapy
(C) Behavioral therapy
(D) Interpersonal therapy

Q482. A patient repeatedly interrupts others during conversation and acts without considering consequences. Which psychological trait does this behavior demonstrate?
(A) Impulsivity
(B) Perseveration
(C) Catatonia
(D) Insight

Q483. A patient describes hearing two voices arguing about their behavior. Which specific hallucination type does this represent?
(A) Running commentary hallucination
(B) Visual hallucination
(C) Tactile hallucination
(D) Command hallucination

Q484. A patient taking antidepressant medication reports sudden agitation, confusion, fever, and muscle rigidity after combining medications. Which syndrome should be suspected?
(A) Acute dystonia
(B) Serotonin syndrome
(C) Neuroleptic malignant syndrome
(D) Hypertensive crisis

Q485. A patient demonstrates difficulty understanding abstract concepts during cognitive testing. Which cognitive domain is impaired?
(A) Abstract reasoning
(B) Orientation
(C) Attention
(D) Memory

Q486. A patient persistently lies about having severe illnesses in order to receive medical attention. Which disorder is most consistent with this behavior?
(A) Conversion disorder
(B) Factitious disorder

(C) Somatic symptom disorder
(D) Illness anxiety disorder

Q487. A patient believes that a famous celebrity is secretly in love with them despite never meeting the person. Which type of delusion is present?
(A) Grandiose delusion
(B) Erotomanic delusion
(C) Somatic delusion
(D) Referential delusion

Q488. A patient repeatedly organizes objects symmetrically and becomes extremely distressed if the arrangement is disturbed. Which disorder is suggested?
(A) Obsessive-compulsive disorder
(B) Adjustment disorder
(C) Hoarding disorder
(D) Body dysmorphic disorder

Q489. A patient experiences sudden episodes of intense fear accompanied by chest pain, dizziness, and shortness of breath. Which condition best explains these symptoms?
(A) Generalized anxiety disorder
(B) Social anxiety disorder
(C) Specific phobia
(D) Panic disorder

Q490. A patient with schizophrenia demonstrates reduced ability to experience pleasure from previously enjoyable activities. Which symptom is this?
(A) Catatonia
(B) Avolition
(C) Anhedonia
(D) Echolalia

Q491. A patient repeatedly echoes the last words spoken by another person during conversation. What phenomenon is this?
(A) Clang association
(B) Perseveration
(C) Echolalia
(D) Neologism

Q492. A patient complains of uncontrollable leg discomfort and an urge to move the legs while resting at night. Which disorder is suggested?
(A) Sleep apnea
(B) Parasomnia
(C) Restless legs syndrome
(D) Narcolepsy

Q493. A patient expresses a fixed belief that their thoughts are being broadcast so others can hear them. Which symptom is this?
(A) Thought blocking
(B) Thought broadcasting
(C) Thought insertion
(D) Thought withdrawal

Q494. A patient repeatedly stores broken items and old newspapers despite having no use for them. What disorder is most consistent with this behavior?
(A) Obsessive-compulsive disorder
(B) Somatic symptom disorder

(C) Hoarding disorder
(D) Panic disorder

Q495. A patient describes feeling emotionally numb and detached after experiencing a traumatic event. Which psychological defense mechanism is this?
(A) Projection
(B) Denial
(C) Regression
(D) Dissociation

Q496. A clinician evaluates a patient's awareness of their mental illness and need for treatment. Which concept is being assessed?
(A) Orientation
(B) Insight
(C) Judgment
(D) Memory

Q497. A patient persistently avoids driving after being involved in a serious accident months earlier. Which behavioral response is this?
(A) Avoidance behavior
(B) Compulsion
(C) Hallucination
(D) Delusion

Q498. A patient demonstrates extremely rapid speech that is difficult to interrupt during a manic episode. What speech characteristic is this?
(A) Echolalia
(B) Tangentiality
(C) Circumstantiality
(D) Pressured speech

Q499. A patient with chronic anxiety reports persistent muscle tension, fatigue, and irritability for several months. Which disorder is most consistent with these symptoms?
(A) Generalized anxiety disorder
(B) Social anxiety disorder
(C) Adjustment disorder
(D) Panic disorder

Q500. A patient expresses feelings of worthlessness and guilt while believing that the world would be better without them. Which cognitive distortion is most evident?
(A) Negative self-evaluation
(B) Overgeneralization
(C) Magical thinking
(D) Catastrophic thinking

Answer Key and Explanation (401-500)

Q401. Answer: B

Explanation: The clinical presentation reflects a classic manic episode characterized by elevated mood, decreased need for sleep, pressured speech, increased activity, and risky behaviors lasting nearly a week. A manic episode is sufficient to establish the diagnosis even if depressive episodes have not occurred. Such episodes involve marked impairment in functioning or require clinical attention due to behavioral consequences. The presence of expansive mood and impulsive behavior strongly suggests a severe mood elevation rather than a mild hypomanic state. Proper recognition is essential because treatment typically requires mood stabilizers or antipsychotics rather than antidepressant therapy alone.

Q402. Answer: C

Explanation: This reaction represents an acute extrapyramidal effect involving involuntary muscle contractions of the neck and face. The condition often appears shortly after initiation or dose increase of certain antipsychotic medications. It results from dopamine blockade in the basal ganglia leading to abnormal muscle tone and spasms. Rapid recognition is important because the reaction can be extremely uncomfortable and frightening for the patient. Prompt treatment with anticholinergic or antihistamine medications typically produces rapid symptom relief.

Q403. Answer: C

Explanation: This tool is designed to screen individuals for depressive symptoms and assess their severity over time. It is widely used in primary care and psychiatric settings to assist clinicians in identifying individuals who may require further evaluation. The questionnaire is brief and aligns with common diagnostic symptom criteria related to mood, sleep, energy, and concentration. It also provides a quantitative score that helps track treatment response across multiple visits. Consistent use of such screening instruments supports standardized and evidence-based mental health assessment practices.

Q404. Answer: C

Explanation: This assessment scale is specifically designed to evaluate the severity of alcohol withdrawal symptoms. It measures multiple physiologic and neurologic signs such as tremor, nausea, sweating, anxiety, and orientation. Scores obtained from the tool guide clinicians in determining the need for medication therapy and monitoring progression. It is frequently used in inpatient detoxification settings to guide benzodiazepine dosing. Consistent monitoring with this scale helps prevent complications such as seizures or delirium tremens.

Q405. Answer: B

Explanation: This symptom reflects a false belief that external events or communications are directed specifically toward the individual. The belief persists despite clear evidence that the interpretation is incorrect. Such experiences are common in psychotic disorders where distorted interpretations of neutral stimuli occur. The individual perceives special meaning in everyday events that others recognize as unrelated. Identification of these symptoms is important because they often require antipsychotic treatment and careful clinical monitoring.

Q406. Answer: D

Explanation: These symptoms suggest possible toxicity associated with mood stabilizer therapy. Monitoring blood concentrations is essential because the medication has a narrow therapeutic range. Early recognition of toxicity allows clinicians to adjust dosing or discontinue therapy before severe neurologic complications occur. Laboratory confirmation guides further management decisions and ensures patient safety. Prompt evaluation prevents progression to severe toxicity involving seizures or altered consciousness.

Q407. Answer: B

Explanation: This treatment approach focuses on the relationship between thoughts, emotions, and behaviors. The therapy aims to identify distorted cognitive patterns that contribute to emotional distress.

Patients learn structured strategies to challenge maladaptive thinking and develop healthier interpretations of events. Behavioral techniques are often combined with cognitive restructuring exercises. The approach is widely supported by research for the treatment of mood and anxiety disorders.

Q408. Answer: A

Explanation: This condition involves a subjective sense of inner restlessness accompanied by repetitive movements such as pacing or shifting weight. It commonly occurs after initiation or dose increase of dopamine-blocking medications. The sensation can be extremely distressing and may increase risk of medication nonadherence. Early recognition is important because symptoms often respond to medication adjustments or adjunctive treatments. Proper management improves patient comfort and adherence to therapy.

Q409. Answer: B

Explanation: Expressions of suicidal intent combined with access to lethal means represent a significant clinical emergency. Immediate evaluation of risk factors such as intent, plan, and protective factors is necessary to determine appropriate intervention. Ensuring safety is the primary responsibility of the clinician in this situation. Interventions may include removing access to lethal means, initiating crisis services, or arranging emergency hospitalization. Early action significantly reduces the likelihood of self-harm.

Q410. Answer: A

Explanation: Chronic anxiety disorders are often associated with dysregulation of several neurochemical systems involved in stress response. Altered activity in inhibitory and excitatory neurotransmitters contributes to heightened physiological arousal and persistent worry. Reduced inhibitory signaling combined with increased sympathetic activation can maintain symptoms of tension and restlessness. These neurobiological mechanisms explain why medications affecting these systems may improve symptoms. Understanding the underlying neurochemistry assists clinicians in selecting appropriate pharmacologic treatments.

Q412. Answer: C

Explanation: This phenomenon involves a sudden interruption in the train of thought that results in an abrupt halt in speech. The individual often reports that the thought simply disappeared or was removed from their mind. It is frequently observed in psychotic disorders where disturbances in thought processes occur. The pause may last several seconds before conversation resumes on a different topic. Identifying this pattern during assessment provides valuable information about underlying cognitive and psychiatric functioning.

Q411. Answer: C

Explanation: This experience involves perceiving sound without an external stimulus. The voices may comment on the individual's actions or conversations and are perceived as real by the person experiencing them. Such perceptions originate internally but are interpreted as coming from outside sources. These symptoms are commonly associated with certain psychotic disorders and can significantly affect daily functioning. Clinical evaluation focuses on understanding the nature, frequency, and emotional impact of the experience to guide treatment.

Q413. Answer: A

Explanation: The diagnostic criteria require that symptoms not only be present but also cause meaningful disruption in daily functioning. Emotional distress alone is insufficient without evidence of social, occupational, or academic impairment. This requirement ensures that normal variations in mood are not mistaken for clinical disorders. Clinicians must carefully evaluate how symptoms affect relationships, work performance, and self-care. Proper assessment prevents overdiagnosis while ensuring individuals who need treatment receive appropriate care.

Q414. Answer: C

Explanation: This rare but serious reaction is associated with dopamine-blocking medications. It is characterized by severe muscle rigidity, elevated body temperature, and autonomic dysfunction. Laboratory abnormalities may include elevated creatine kinase due to muscle breakdown. Rapid recognition is essential because the condition can progress to life-threatening complications. Treatment typically involves immediate discontinuation of the offending medication and supportive medical management.

Q415. Answer: C

Explanation: This condition is characterized by emotional instability and difficulties in interpersonal relationships. Individuals often experience rapid mood shifts, impulsive behavior, and a chronic sense of emptiness. Fear of abandonment frequently leads to intense and unstable attachments. Self-image may fluctuate dramatically, contributing to interpersonal conflict. Psychotherapeutic interventions that focus on emotional regulation and interpersonal effectiveness are commonly recommended.

Q416. Answer: A

Explanation: This clinical tool measures the severity of symptoms associated with opioid withdrawal. It evaluates physiological and subjective indicators such as heart rate, pupil size, sweating, restlessness, and gastrointestinal discomfort. The resulting score helps clinicians determine appropriate treatment strategies and medication dosing. It is widely used in detoxification and addiction treatment settings. Consistent monitoring allows providers to track progress and adjust interventions accordingly.

Q417. Answer: A

Explanation: This phenomenon involves the perception of sound in the absence of an external auditory stimulus. Individuals may hear voices that speak to them directly or discuss their behavior. Such experiences are common in psychotic disorders and may cause significant distress. The content and frequency of these perceptions are important factors to assess during psychiatric evaluation. Effective treatment often involves antipsychotic medication combined with supportive therapy.

Q418. Answer: A

Explanation: This syndrome occurs when excessive serotonergic activity develops within the central nervous system. It can arise from combining medications that increase serotonin levels. Symptoms frequently include neuromuscular hyperactivity, altered mental status, and autonomic instability. Early identification is important because severe cases may progress rapidly and require urgent treatment. Management typically involves discontinuation of contributing medications and supportive care.

Q419. Answer: C

Explanation: This communication style involves overinclusion of irrelevant details before finally reaching the intended point. Although the conversation becomes lengthy and indirect, the speaker ultimately answers the question. The pattern may occur in several psychiatric conditions including mood disorders and anxiety states. Careful observation of speech patterns provides insight into cognitive organization. Clinicians often redirect the conversation gently to maintain focus during assessment.

Q420. Answer: C

Explanation: This disorder involves chronic depressive symptoms lasting for an extended period. The symptoms are typically less severe than those seen in major depressive episodes but persist for years. Individuals often experience ongoing low mood accompanied by fatigue, low motivation, and poor self-confidence. The prolonged duration distinguishes it from episodic depressive conditions. Treatment frequently involves a combination of psychotherapy and pharmacologic interventions.

Q421. Answer: B

Explanation: This approach focuses on modifying maladaptive behaviors through structured interventions. Techniques such as relaxation training and exposure are designed to reduce anxiety responses. By practicing these skills, individuals gradually learn to control physiological reactions to stress. The therapy emphasizes measurable behavioral change rather than exploration of unconscious conflicts. Research demonstrates strong effectiveness of these strategies for anxiety-related conditions.

Q422. Answer: D

Explanation: This evaluation determines whether an individual can make informed decisions regarding medical care. The assessment focuses on the ability to comprehend relevant information and consider potential outcomes. Patients must demonstrate reasoning about choices and clearly express their preferences. Capacity is task specific and may fluctuate depending on clinical conditions. Determining this ability ensures that ethical standards of autonomy and informed consent are upheld.

Q423. Answer: C

Explanation: This movement disorder results from dopamine receptor blockade in motor pathways of the brain. Symptoms resemble those seen in degenerative neurologic conditions affecting movement. Patients may exhibit slowed movements, stiffness, and tremors. The condition usually develops within weeks of initiating certain medications. Adjusting therapy or using medications that restore neurotransmitter balance can help relieve symptoms.

Q424. Answer: C

Explanation: This psychological framework emphasizes the role of unconscious processes in shaping behavior and emotional experience. Treatment involves exploring early life experiences and unresolved internal conflicts. The therapeutic relationship provides a setting for examining patterns that influence present behavior. Insight gained through reflection is believed to facilitate psychological change. Although less commonly used alone today, its concepts influence many modern therapeutic approaches.

Q425. Answer: C

Explanation: Panic symptoms involve activation of brain circuits related to the stress response. Neurochemical changes affecting serotonin and norepinephrine pathways influence emotional regulation and autonomic arousal. Dysregulation within these systems contributes to sudden episodes of overwhelming fear. Medications targeting these neurotransmitters are commonly used to reduce symptom frequency. Psychotherapy focusing on cognitive restructuring and exposure can also improve outcomes.

Q426. Answer: D

Explanation: Long-term exposure to certain medications can lead the body to adapt to their presence. When the medication is suddenly discontinued, the nervous system may become overactive. This physiological adaptation results in withdrawal symptoms that can range from mild discomfort to serious complications. Gradual tapering of the medication helps prevent these effects. Understanding this concept guides safe prescribing and discontinuation practices.

Q427. Answer: B

Explanation: This perception involves experiencing a smell without an external stimulus present. Such sensations may occur in several psychiatric or neurologic conditions. They can also be associated with seizure activity or certain brain lesions. Careful clinical evaluation is necessary to determine the underlying cause. Identifying sensory disturbances helps guide diagnostic investigation and treatment planning.

Q428. Answer: B

Explanation: This disorder involves intrusive thoughts that create significant anxiety. Individuals perform repetitive behaviors or mental acts in an attempt to reduce distress. These behaviors are often excessive and time-consuming. The individual usually recognizes that the actions are unreasonable but feels compelled to perform them. Treatment often involves cognitive behavioral therapy combined with medications that affect serotonin regulation.

Q429. Answer: A

Explanation: This experience reflects a disturbance in the sense of ownership over one's thoughts. Individuals believe that thoughts originate from outside sources rather than their own mind. The symptom is commonly associated with psychotic disorders involving severe disruption in perception of reality. It may contribute to significant distress and impairment in functioning. Recognition of this symptom assists clinicians in making accurate diagnostic assessments.

Q430. Answer: B
Explanation: This condition is characterized by an acute disturbance in attention and awareness that develops rapidly. Cognitive changes often fluctuate throughout the day and may include memory impairment or perceptual disturbances. The syndrome is commonly associated with medical illness, medication effects, or metabolic abnormalities. Early identification is important because the underlying cause is often reversible. Prompt treatment focuses on addressing the precipitating medical condition.

Q431. Answer: A
Explanation: These manifestations involve a reduction or absence of normal emotional and behavioral functions. Individuals may show flat facial expressions, decreased verbal communication, and limited engagement in daily activities. Such symptoms are often associated with impaired motivation and social withdrawal. They tend to persist even when hallucinations or delusions improve. Effective management often requires long-term therapeutic strategies including psychosocial interventions and medication support.

Q432. Answer: B
Explanation: This pattern involves early morning awakening with difficulty returning to sleep. It is commonly associated with depressive disorders and reflects disruptions in circadian rhythm regulation. Patients often describe feeling exhausted despite spending many hours in bed. The symptom may worsen mood disturbances and impair daytime functioning. Recognition of sleep patterns helps clinicians evaluate severity and treatment response in mood disorders.

Q433. Answer: B
Explanation: This severe withdrawal complication occurs after prolonged heavy alcohol consumption. It typically begins several days after cessation and includes confusion, agitation, tremors, and hallucinations. Autonomic instability such as tachycardia and hypertension is common. Without prompt medical treatment the condition can become life threatening. Management requires close monitoring and pharmacologic intervention to stabilize symptoms.

Q434. Answer: B
Explanation: This experience involves a sense of separation from one's own body or mental processes. Individuals may feel as though they are observing themselves from an external perspective. Reality testing generally remains intact despite the unusual perception. The symptom is often associated with severe anxiety, trauma, or dissociative conditions. Proper evaluation helps distinguish it from psychotic experiences.

Q435. Answer: B
Explanation: This behavioral strategy involves systematic confrontation with feared stimuli. The process occurs gradually so the patient can develop tolerance and reduce avoidance behaviors. Repeated exposure allows the brain to learn that the feared situation is not dangerous. Over time anxiety responses diminish through habituation. This method is considered highly effective for treating many anxiety disorders.

Q436. Answer: D
Explanation: This pattern involves rapid transitions between loosely related ideas. Speech may appear pressured and difficult to interrupt. The individual often moves from one concept to another based on superficial associations. It is commonly observed in manic states where thought processes accelerate dramatically. Recognizing this pattern helps clinicians assess mood disorders.

Q437. Answer: D
Explanation: This rare but potentially fatal complication involves a dangerous reduction in white blood cells. The condition weakens the immune system and increases susceptibility to severe infections. Because early symptoms may be subtle, regular laboratory monitoring is mandatory. Blood testing allows clinicians to detect abnormalities before severe complications occur. Adherence to monitoring guidelines ensures safe use of this medication.

Q438. Answer: D
Explanation: The distressing motor restlessness experienced by some patients can be alleviated with medications that reduce sympathetic nervous system activity. These agents help calm physical agitation and reduce uncomfortable internal sensations. They are commonly used when dose adjustments alone do not relieve symptoms. Treatment improves patient comfort and helps maintain adherence to psychiatric medication. Effective management reduces the risk of treatment discontinuation.
Q439. Answer: A
Explanation: This belief involves the conviction that others intend to harm or conspire against the individual. The perception persists despite lack of evidence and often causes significant distress. Such beliefs can lead to fear, mistrust, and social withdrawal. They are frequently observed in psychotic disorders. Careful evaluation and treatment are necessary to address distorted interpretations of reality.
Q440. Answer: A
Explanation: This behavior involves the involuntary imitation of another person's physical actions. It may occur in certain psychiatric and neurologic conditions. The phenomenon reflects disturbances in motor control and behavioral regulation. Observing such behaviors during assessment can provide valuable diagnostic clues. Identification helps guide further evaluation and management.
Q441. Answer: C
Explanation: This condition is characterized by intense fear of negative evaluation in social or performance situations. Individuals may avoid gatherings, conversations, or public activities due to anxiety about embarrassment. The avoidance can significantly impair occupational and social functioning. Physical symptoms such as sweating, trembling, and rapid heartbeat often accompany the fear. Psychotherapy and pharmacologic treatments are effective in reducing symptoms.
Q442. Answer: B
Explanation: This behavior occurs when individuals unconsciously create information to compensate for memory loss. The person genuinely believes the invented details to be accurate. It often appears in neurocognitive disorders where memory retrieval is impaired. The process differs from intentional lying because the individual lacks awareness of the inaccuracy. Understanding this phenomenon helps clinicians assess cognitive impairment.
Q443. Answer: C
Explanation: Certain antidepressant medications can affect neurotransmitter pathways involved in sexual function. Changes in serotonin activity may interfere with arousal and orgasmic response. These effects are relatively common and may affect treatment adherence. Clinicians should discuss potential side effects openly with patients. Adjusting medication or dosage can sometimes improve symptoms while maintaining therapeutic benefit.
Q444. Answer: B
Explanation: This condition involves excessive concern about having or developing a serious illness. Individuals remain preoccupied with health-related fears even when medical examinations show no disease. The anxiety may lead to frequent checking behaviors or repeated medical consultations. Distress persists despite reassurance from healthcare providers. Treatment often focuses on cognitive behavioral strategies to reduce health-related anxiety.
Q445. Answer: B
Explanation: This movement disorder develops after prolonged exposure to dopamine-blocking medications. It involves involuntary, repetitive movements of the face, mouth, and tongue. The symptoms may persist even after medication adjustments. Early detection is important because the condition can become permanent if untreated. Monitoring patients regularly helps identify early signs and guide medication changes.
Q446. Answer: A

Explanation: This condition involves excessive fear or distress related to separation from attachment figures. The anxiety is disproportionate to the individual's developmental level. Symptoms may include persistent worry about losing loved ones or being alone. Avoidance behaviors and physical complaints can occur when separation is anticipated. Recognition of these patterns assists clinicians in planning appropriate therapy.

Q447. Answer: B

Explanation: Emotional distress after the loss of a loved one is a natural psychological response. Individuals may experience sadness, sleep disturbances, and reduced interest in activities. These reactions generally lessen over time as the person adapts to the loss. Support from family, friends, and counseling often helps facilitate coping. Clinicians must distinguish this normal process from more severe mood disorders requiring medical treatment.

Q448. Answer: C

Explanation: This therapeutic model focuses on recognizing and developing an individual's existing abilities and resources. Rather than concentrating solely on problems, the approach highlights positive attributes. Encouraging patients to utilize their strengths can improve confidence and adaptive functioning. The process promotes resilience in managing stress and adversity. Many modern recovery-oriented mental health programs incorporate this philosophy.

Q449. Answer: C

Explanation: This experience occurs when a real external stimulus is misinterpreted by the brain. The perception is based on an actual object or event but is inaccurately perceived. Such misinterpretations can occur when lighting is poor or attention is impaired. Once the stimulus is clarified the person typically recognizes the mistake. Understanding these phenomena helps differentiate perceptual disturbances during mental status examinations.

Q450. Answer: C

Explanation: This therapeutic approach was developed to help individuals manage severe emotional dysregulation. It combines cognitive behavioral techniques with mindfulness practices. Skills training focuses on distress tolerance, emotional regulation, interpersonal effectiveness, and mindfulness. The therapy is particularly beneficial for individuals with chronic emotional instability. Structured sessions and skills practice help patients develop healthier coping strategies.

Q451. Answer: A

Explanation: This pattern includes mood reactivity combined with specific biological symptoms. Individuals often experience excessive sleeping, increased appetite, and sensitivity to interpersonal rejection. The presentation differs from other depressive subtypes that involve insomnia and loss of appetite. Recognition of symptom patterns helps guide treatment decisions. Certain medications may be particularly effective for this subtype.

Q452. Answer: A

Explanation: Mood regulation involves complex interactions among several neurotransmitter pathways. Changes in these chemical messengers influence emotional stability and energy levels. Dysregulation within these systems contributes to both manic and depressive phases. Pharmacologic treatments often target these neurotransmitters to stabilize mood. Understanding neurobiology supports effective medication selection and management.

Q453. Answer: B

Explanation: This condition involves recurrent urges to pull out one's own hair. The behavior often leads to visible hair loss and emotional distress. Individuals may attempt to resist the impulse but feel increasing tension beforehand. Relief or gratification typically occurs after the behavior. Behavioral therapy approaches are commonly used to help reduce the repetitive action.

Q454. Answer: C

Explanation: This belief involves false convictions about bodily functions or physical health. Individuals may insist that their body is diseased or damaged despite normal medical findings. Such ideas persist even when clear evidence contradicts them. These beliefs can cause significant anxiety and repeated medical consultations. Accurate identification assists clinicians in diagnosing underlying psychiatric conditions.

Q455. Answer: C

Explanation: This set of mental processes allows individuals to plan, organize, and regulate goal-directed behavior. Damage to brain regions responsible for these functions can impair problem solving and decision making. Individuals may struggle with initiating tasks or managing multiple steps in an activity. Such deficits significantly affect independence and daily functioning. Rehabilitation strategies often focus on improving these higher-level cognitive abilities.

Q456. Answer: C

Explanation: This practice involves intentionally directing attention to the present moment. Individuals learn to observe thoughts and sensations without reacting impulsively or critically. Regular practice can reduce stress and improve emotional regulation. The technique is widely used in modern psychotherapeutic approaches. It promotes greater awareness of internal experiences and enhances psychological well-being.

Q457. Answer: D

Explanation: This condition develops following exposure to a traumatic event involving actual or threatened harm. Individuals may experience intrusive memories, nightmares, and persistent hyperarousal. Avoidance of reminders related to the trauma is common. Symptoms lasting longer than one month suggest a chronic trauma-related condition. Early recognition allows timely psychological intervention and support.

Q458. Answer: A

Explanation: This condition involves ongoing difficulty initiating or maintaining sleep. Psychological factors such as anxiety and excessive worry often contribute to the problem. Individuals frequently experience daytime fatigue and impaired concentration. Poor sleep quality may worsen underlying mental health conditions. Behavioral strategies and sleep hygiene practices are common components of treatment.

Q459. Answer: D

Explanation: This condition involves persistent difficulty discarding possessions regardless of their actual value. The accumulation of items can clutter living spaces and interfere with daily activities. Individuals often experience strong emotional attachment to objects. Attempts to remove items may cause significant distress. Therapeutic interventions typically focus on decision-making skills and gradual decluttering strategies.

Q460. Answer: B

Explanation: This principle emphasizes understanding and respecting diverse cultural backgrounds in healthcare delivery. Clinicians recognize that beliefs, traditions, and social factors influence health behaviors. Incorporating these perspectives improves communication and patient trust. It also ensures that treatment recommendations are appropriate and acceptable to the individual. Such awareness supports equitable and effective mental health care.

Q461. Answer: A

Explanation: This medication has a narrow therapeutic range and requires regular monitoring to prevent toxicity. Blood concentrations help clinicians ensure that levels remain within a safe and effective range. Elevated levels may produce neurological and gastrointestinal symptoms. Regular monitoring also allows dosage adjustments based on renal function and clinical response. Maintaining therapeutic levels improves mood stabilization while reducing the risk of adverse effects.

Q462. Answer: D

Explanation: This condition involves marked disturbances in motor behavior and responsiveness. Individuals may remain motionless or maintain unusual postures for extended periods. Speech may be absent or extremely limited during episodes. The syndrome can occur in several psychiatric and medical conditions. Early recognition is essential because treatment may require specific pharmacologic or medical interventions.

Q463. Answer: D

Explanation: This neurological sleep disorder involves abnormal regulation of sleep-wake cycles. Sudden muscle weakness episodes may occur during strong emotional experiences. Individuals often experience overwhelming daytime sleepiness despite adequate nighttime rest. These episodes may interfere with work, school, or social activities. Diagnosis often requires specialized sleep studies and clinical evaluation.

Q464. Answer: B

Explanation: This belief involves an exaggerated sense of importance, power, or identity. Individuals may believe they have unique abilities or a special role in the world. These convictions remain fixed even when clearly unrealistic. Such beliefs are often observed in mood or psychotic disorders. Careful assessment helps determine appropriate treatment strategies.

Q465. Answer: B

Explanation: This behavior represents repetitive actions performed to reduce anxiety caused by intrusive thoughts. Individuals feel driven to perform the behavior even though they recognize it may be excessive. The act temporarily relieves distress but reinforces the cycle of obsession and ritual. Over time the pattern becomes increasingly difficult to control. Behavioral therapy techniques are commonly used to interrupt this cycle.

Q466. Answer: C

Explanation: This disorder involves intense fear of situations where escape might be difficult or help unavailable. Individuals may avoid public spaces, transportation, or crowded environments. The fear is often linked to previous panic experiences. Avoidance behaviors can significantly restrict daily functioning and independence. Treatment often includes psychotherapy and medications to reduce anxiety symptoms.

Q467. Answer: D

Explanation: This therapy emphasizes emotional regulation, distress tolerance, and interpersonal effectiveness. Structured skills training helps individuals manage impulsive reactions and intense emotions. Mindfulness techniques are integrated to increase awareness of emotional triggers. The approach has demonstrated effectiveness for individuals with severe emotional instability. Long-term participation improves coping strategies and relationship functioning.

Q468. Answer: A

Explanation: This pattern refers to predictable changes in mood at different times of the day. Some individuals experience the most severe symptoms during early morning hours. Energy and mood may gradually improve later in the day. Such variations are often associated with certain depressive subtypes. Observing these patterns helps clinicians better understand symptom progression.

Q469. Answer: D

Explanation: This phenomenon occurs when individuals invent new words or phrases that are not recognized in normal language. The newly created terms may have personal meaning but are not understood by others. It is commonly observed in severe thought disorders. The speech pattern reflects disorganized thinking and impaired communication. Recognition of such features helps clinicians assess severity of psychosis.

Q470. Answer: A

Explanation: This pattern involves persistent repetition of words, phrases, or ideas. The response continues even when the conversation topic changes. It may occur in several neurological or psychiatric conditions affecting cognitive flexibility. The behavior reflects difficulty shifting attention or thought processes. Identifying such patterns provides insight into underlying cognitive dysfunction.

Q471. Answer: A

Explanation: This disorder involves a cluster of emotional, cognitive, and physical symptoms lasting at least two weeks. Individuals experience depressed mood along with reduced pleasure in daily activities. Sleep disturbances, appetite changes, and fatigue commonly accompany the condition. Symptoms significantly affect social and occupational functioning. Early diagnosis allows timely treatment through psychotherapy and medication.

Q472. Answer: A

Explanation: This response involves a disruption in the normal integration of thoughts, emotions, and memories. Individuals may detach from distressing experiences as a protective mechanism. Emotional numbing and avoidance are common features following traumatic events. Although protective initially, persistent dissociation can interfere with recovery. Therapeutic interventions focus on safely processing traumatic memories.

Q473. Answer: A

Explanation: This assessment measures short-term memory and the ability to retain new information. The patient must encode, store, and retrieve information within a brief interval. Difficulties performing this task may indicate cognitive impairment or neurological dysfunction. Memory testing is a key component of mental status examinations. Results help guide further diagnostic evaluation.

Q474. Answer: A

Explanation: This experience involves a distorted perception of the external environment. Individuals may describe surroundings as foggy, artificial, or unreal. Despite these perceptions, they typically recognize that the feeling is subjective. The phenomenon often occurs during severe anxiety or traumatic stress. Proper assessment helps differentiate it from psychotic disorders.

Q475. Answer: B

Explanation: These medications help regulate abnormal fluctuations in mood. They are commonly used to prevent both manic and depressive episodes. Treatment aims to maintain emotional stability over long periods. Regular monitoring may be required to ensure safe and effective dosing. Combining medication with psychotherapy often improves long-term outcomes.

Q476. Answer: A

Explanation: This feature involves intrusive and persistent thoughts that cause significant anxiety. Individuals attempt to neutralize the distress by performing repetitive behaviors. The cycle of intrusive thoughts and ritualized actions can become time consuming. The person often recognizes that the fears are excessive but struggles to resist them. Cognitive behavioral interventions are frequently used to treat these patterns.

Q477. Answer: C

Explanation: This phenomenon refers to worsening confusion and agitation during evening hours. Individuals with cognitive impairment may experience increased restlessness or wandering. Changes in lighting and fatigue may contribute to this pattern. Caregivers often report behavioral disturbances occurring late in the day. Environmental adjustments and structured routines may help reduce symptoms.

Q478. Answer: C

Explanation: This disorder involves chronic and excessive worry about multiple aspects of life. The anxiety is difficult to control and persists for long periods. Individuals often experience fatigue, muscle tension, irritability, and sleep disturbance. Symptoms significantly interfere with concentration and daily functioning. Treatment typically includes psychotherapy and medications targeting anxiety regulation.

Q479. Answer: C

Explanation: These difficulties involve impaired mental processes necessary for learning and decision making. Problems with attention and memory can interfere with daily functioning. Individuals may struggle with planning tasks or solving problems. Such deficits often persist even when other symptoms improve. Cognitive rehabilitation strategies may help enhance functioning.

Q480. Answer: A

Explanation: This pattern involves recurrent depressive episodes linked to specific seasons. Reduced sunlight exposure during colder months may influence biological rhythms. Individuals often experience fatigue, increased sleep, and changes in appetite. Symptoms typically resolve as daylight hours increase. Light therapy and antidepressant treatment are common management strategies.

Q481. Answer: D

Explanation: This therapeutic approach focuses on the connection between mood symptoms and social relationships. The therapist works with the patient to identify communication patterns and interpersonal conflicts. Improving relationship skills can reduce emotional distress and enhance support systems. The therapy is structured and time limited. Research supports its effectiveness for treating mood disorders.

Q482. Answer: A

Explanation: This characteristic involves acting quickly without adequate reflection or planning. Individuals may struggle to delay gratification or consider long-term outcomes. The behavior can lead to risky decisions and interpersonal difficulties. Impulsivity is often observed in several psychiatric conditions. Treatment focuses on developing self-control and coping strategies.

Q483. Answer: A

Explanation: This experience involves voices discussing the person's actions or thoughts. The voices may provide commentary as events occur. Such symptoms are frequently associated with psychotic disorders. The phenomenon can be distressing and interfere with concentration. Effective treatment usually involves antipsychotic medication and supportive therapy.

Q484. Answer: B

Explanation: This condition occurs when excessive serotonin activity develops within the nervous system. It often results from combining medications that increase serotonin levels. Symptoms include mental status changes, neuromuscular abnormalities, and autonomic instability. The syndrome can progress rapidly if not recognized early. Immediate discontinuation of contributing medications is necessary.

Q485. Answer: A

Explanation: This mental ability involves interpreting complex ideas and identifying relationships between concepts. Individuals with impairment may struggle to explain proverbs or recognize similarities between objects. The deficit may occur in several neurological or psychiatric conditions. Assessing abstract thinking helps evaluate higher level cognitive functioning. Results contribute to comprehensive mental status examination findings.

Q486. Answer: B

Explanation: This condition involves intentionally producing or exaggerating symptoms without obvious external rewards. The primary motivation is to assume the sick role and receive attention or care. Unlike malingering, the behavior is not driven by financial or legal incentives. Individuals may undergo numerous medical procedures unnecessarily. Psychological evaluation is essential to identify underlying motivations.

Q487. Answer: B

Explanation: This belief involves the conviction that another person is romantically interested in the individual. The supposed admirer is often someone of higher social status or public prominence. The belief persists even when there is no contact or evidence supporting it. Such delusions can lead to repeated attempts to communicate with the imagined admirer. Careful assessment is required to ensure safety and appropriate treatment.

Q488. Answer: A

Explanation: This condition involves intrusive thoughts and repetitive behaviors performed to reduce anxiety. The individual feels compelled to arrange or order objects in a specific manner. Distress occurs when the pattern is disrupted. Such behaviors can consume significant time and interfere with daily functioning. Treatment often includes behavioral therapy focused on exposure and response prevention.

Q489. Answer: D

Explanation: This disorder involves recurrent, unexpected episodes of intense anxiety known as panic attacks. Symptoms often include palpitations, sweating, trembling, and feelings of impending doom. Episodes usually peak within minutes and may occur without clear triggers. Many individuals begin to fear future attacks and change their behavior accordingly. Effective treatment includes psychotherapy and pharmacologic therapy.

Q490. Answer: C

Explanation: This symptom refers to diminished capacity to experience pleasure or interest in activities. Individuals may withdraw from hobbies, relationships, or social events. The change reflects disruptions in brain systems involved in reward processing. It commonly occurs in several mood and psychotic disorders. Recognizing this feature helps clinicians evaluate emotional functioning.

Q491. Answer: C

Explanation: This speech disturbance involves automatic repetition of another person's words. It may occur immediately after hearing the phrase or sentence. The behavior is often associated with certain neurological or psychiatric conditions. Communication becomes limited because the individual does not generate independent responses. Observing this pattern during assessment provides useful diagnostic information.

Q492. Answer: C

Explanation: This condition involves unpleasant sensations in the legs accompanied by an urge to move them. Symptoms typically worsen during periods of inactivity or at night. Movement temporarily relieves the discomfort. Sleep disruption and daytime fatigue often occur. Evaluation may include assessment of iron levels and neurological function.

Q493. Answer: B

Explanation: This experience involves the belief that one's thoughts are accessible to others. Individuals may feel that private mental activity is no longer hidden. The symptom represents a disturbance in the perception of personal boundaries. It is commonly associated with psychotic disorders. Identifying such beliefs assists clinicians in diagnostic assessment.

Q494. Answer: C

Explanation: This condition involves persistent difficulty discarding possessions regardless of their value. The accumulation of objects can lead to cluttered living spaces. Emotional attachment to items makes discarding them extremely distressing. Over time the environment may become unsafe or unsanitary. Treatment often includes cognitive behavioral strategies focusing on decision making and organization.

Q495. Answer: D

Explanation: This coping response involves separation of thoughts, emotions, or memories from conscious awareness. It may develop as a protective mechanism during overwhelming stress. Emotional numbing and detachment can temporarily reduce psychological distress. However persistent dissociation may interfere with emotional processing. Therapeutic approaches focus on safely integrating traumatic experiences.

Q496. Answer: B

Explanation: This concept refers to the degree to which individuals recognize their condition and understand its implications. Some patients may fully acknowledge their symptoms while others deny illness entirely. Insight influences treatment adherence and willingness to engage in care. Evaluating this dimension is a standard component of psychiatric assessment. Improved awareness often develops gradually during recovery.

Q497. Answer: A

Explanation: This response involves deliberately staying away from situations associated with fear or trauma. Avoidance may temporarily reduce anxiety but prevents emotional processing of the event. Over time the behavior can limit normal functioning and independence. Such patterns are commonly seen in trauma-related disorders. Therapeutic strategies often include gradual exposure to feared situations.

Q498. Answer: D

Explanation: This communication pattern involves accelerated speech driven by heightened energy and excitement. The individual may speak continuously and resist interruptions. Thoughts often move quickly, making conversation difficult to follow. It commonly appears during manic episodes. Recognition of this feature assists clinicians in identifying mood elevation.

Q499. Answer: A

Explanation: This condition involves long-term excessive worry about everyday situations. The anxiety is difficult to control and occurs on most days. Physical symptoms often include muscle tension, restlessness, and fatigue. Sleep disturbance and difficulty concentrating are also common. Treatment usually involves psychotherapy combined with medications that reduce anxiety.

Q500. Answer: A

Explanation: This pattern involves harsh and unrealistic judgments about oneself. Individuals may interpret normal setbacks as evidence of personal failure. Persistent negative beliefs contribute to depressive symptoms and low self-esteem. Such cognitive distortions influence emotional reactions and behavior. Cognitive restructuring techniques are often used to challenge and modify these beliefs.

Question (501-600)

Q501. A patient with schizophrenia withdraws from social interactions and shows minimal interest in daily activities. Which negative symptom is most consistent with this behavior?

(A) Delusion
(B) Avolition
(C) Echolalia
(D) Hallucination

Q502. A patient suddenly becomes frightened and reports seeing a snake on the floor, but further inspection reveals it is only a rope. What type of perceptual disturbance occurred?

(A) Confabulation
(B) Hallucination
(C) Illusion
(D) Delusion

Q503. A patient demonstrates excessive talking, inflated self-esteem, decreased need for sleep, and risky decision making. These symptoms are most consistent with which mood episode?

(A) Hypomanic episode
(B) Depressive episode
(C) Manic episode
(D) Mixed episode

Q504. A patient persistently fears that their body emits a foul odor despite reassurance from others that no odor exists. Which disorder is suggested?

(A) Illness anxiety disorder
(B) Delusional disorder
(C) Body dysmorphic disorder
(D) Panic disorder

Q505. A patient receiving antidepressant therapy reports improved mood but experiences excessive sweating and tremors after combining medications. Which neurotransmitter excess is responsible?

(A) Acetylcholine
(B) Dopamine
(C) Serotonin
(D) Histamine

Q506. A clinician asks a patient to interpret the proverb "People in glass houses should not throw stones." Which cognitive ability is being assessed?

(A) Abstract thinking
(B) Immediate memory
(C) Orientation
(D) Attention

Q507. A patient repeatedly washes hands after touching everyday objects because of intrusive contamination fears. Which behavioral therapy technique is most effective for this condition?

(A) Free association
(B) Hypnosis
(C) Systematic desensitization
(D) Exposure and response prevention

Q508. A patient becomes extremely anxious when entering elevators or enclosed spaces. Which disorder most closely matches this fear?

(A) Panic disorder
(B) Agoraphobia

(C) Social anxiety disorder
(D) Specific phobia

Q509. A patient insists that strangers are placing harmful chemicals into their food. Which type of delusion is present?
(A) Referential delusion
(B) Persecutory delusion
(C) Somatic delusion
(D) Grandiose delusion

Q510. A patient suddenly stops speaking mid-sentence and appears unable to continue their train of thought. Which thought disturbance is this?
(A) Flight of ideas
(B) Circumstantiality
(C) Thought blocking
(D) Tangentiality

Q511. A patient demonstrates persistent sadness accompanied by slowed movements and reduced speech. Which psychomotor change is present?
(A) Catatonia
(B) Psychomotor retardation
(C) Psychomotor agitation
(D) Hyperactivity

Q512. A patient frequently complains about multiple physical symptoms but medical tests reveal no identifiable cause. Which disorder is suggested?
(A) Social anxiety disorder
(B) Bipolar disorder
(C) Panic disorder
(D) Somatic symptom disorder

Q513. A patient repeatedly imitates another person's speech during conversation. Which phenomenon is this?
(A) Echolalia
(B) Clang association
(C) Neologism
(D) Perseveration

Q514. A patient reports feeling excessively energetic and sleeping only three hours per night without fatigue. Which symptom is most characteristic of manic states?
(A) Social withdrawal
(B) Excessive appetite
(C) Decreased need for sleep
(D) Memory impairment

Q515. A patient expresses strong fear of gaining weight despite being significantly underweight. Which eating disorder is most consistent with this presentation?
(A) Anorexia nervosa
(B) Binge eating disorder
(C) Bulimia nervosa
(D) Avoidant eating disorder

Q516. A patient repeatedly engages in binge eating followed by self-induced vomiting. Which eating disorder does this behavior indicate?
(A) Anorexia nervosa
(B) Binge eating disorder

(C) Bulimia nervosa
(D) Avoidant restrictive disorder

Q517. A patient frequently blames others for their own mistakes and refuses to accept responsibility. Which defense mechanism is most evident?
(A) Regression
(B) Displacement
(C) Sublimation
(D) Projection

Q518. A patient becomes hostile toward coworkers after receiving criticism from a supervisor. Which defense mechanism explains redirecting anger toward others?
(A) Rationalization
(B) Denial
(C) Reaction formation
(D) Displacement

Q519. A patient laughs while describing a tragic event that occurred recently. Which defense mechanism is this?
(A) Denial
(B) Intellectualization
(C) Incongruent affect
(D) Reaction formation

Q520. A patient experiences brief episodes of paralysis when falling asleep or waking. Which sleep phenomenon is described?
(A) Sleep apnea
(B) Insomnia
(C) Sleep paralysis
(D) Narcolepsy

Q521. A patient persistently worries about their job performance despite positive feedback from supervisors. Which cognitive distortion is this?
(A) Catastrophizing
(B) Personalization
(C) Overgeneralization
(D) All-or-nothing thinking

Q522. A patient with dementia frequently becomes confused about the date and location. Which cognitive domain is impaired?
(A) Insight
(B) Judgment
(C) Orientation
(D) Abstraction

Q523. A patient insists that their neighbors are sending them secret coded messages through hand gestures. Which symptom does this represent?
(A) Grandiose delusion
(B) Nihilistic delusion
(C) Somatic delusion
(D) Delusion of reference

Q524. A patient describes hearing a voice instructing them to harm themselves. What type of hallucination is this?
(A) Command hallucination
(B) Tactile hallucination

(C) Visual hallucination
(D) Olfactory hallucination

Q525. A patient has difficulty maintaining attention during a conversation and frequently becomes distracted. Which cognitive function is impaired?

(A) Orientation
(B) Memory
(C) Language
(D) Attention

Q526. A patient develops tremors, sweating, nausea, and anxiety several hours after stopping heavy alcohol use. What condition is most likely present?

(A) Alcohol poisoning
(B) Alcohol intoxication
(C) Alcohol withdrawal
(D) Delirium tremens

Q527. A patient begins pacing continuously and reports feeling extremely restless after starting a new medication. Which adverse effect is occurring?

(A) Akathisia
(B) Tardive dyskinesia
(C) Catatonia
(D) Acute dystonia

Q528. A patient reports hearing music playing despite no external sound source. Which perceptual disturbance is present?

(A) Confabulation
(B) Auditory hallucination
(C) Illusion
(D) Delusion

Q529. A patient becomes extremely anxious when speaking in public due to fear of embarrassment. Which disorder best explains this behavior?

(A) Social anxiety disorder
(B) Generalized anxiety disorder
(C) Panic disorder
(D) Specific phobia

Q530. A patient suddenly develops muscle rigidity and high fever after receiving antipsychotic medication. Which life-threatening condition should be suspected?

(A) Serotonin syndrome
(B) Acute dystonia
(C) Hypertensive crisis
(D) Neuroleptic malignant syndrome

Q531. A patient consistently arrives late to appointments because they underestimate how long tasks will take. Which executive function deficit is most evident?

(A) Language comprehension
(B) Time management
(C) Sensory processing
(D) Visual perception

Q532. A patient avoids leaving home due to fear that panic symptoms may occur in public places. Which condition is most consistent with this pattern?

(A) Specific phobia
(B) Panic disorder

(C) Separation anxiety disorder
(D) Agoraphobia

Q533. A patient begins talking rapidly and rhyming words that sound similar rather than expressing meaningful ideas. Which speech pattern is this?
(A) Echolalia
(B) Neologism
(C) Clang association
(D) Perseveration

Q534. A patient reports feeling detached from reality and perceiving the world as foggy or unreal. Which phenomenon is this?
(A) Illusion
(B) Derealization
(C) Depersonalization
(D) Hallucination

Q535. A patient insists that their internal organs have stopped functioning even though medical tests are normal. Which delusional theme is present?
(A) Referential delusion
(B) Erotomanic delusion
(C) Nihilistic delusion
(D) Grandiose delusion

Q536. A patient repeatedly pulls hair from their scalp resulting in noticeable hair loss. Which disorder is most consistent with this behavior?
(A) Illness anxiety disorder
(B) Body dysmorphic disorder
(C) Hoarding disorder
(D) Trichotillomania

Q537. A patient suddenly begins speaking incoherently with disorganized word combinations that lack grammatical structure. Which speech disturbance is this?
(A) Circumstantiality
(B) Echolalia
(C) Word salad
(D) Perseveration

Q538. A patient displays extreme fear of snakes and avoids parks or nature trails where snakes might be present. Which disorder does this behavior represent?
(A) Social anxiety disorder
(B) Panic disorder
(C) Specific phobia
(D) Generalized anxiety disorder

Q539. A patient insists that they are responsible for controlling the weather through their thoughts. Which type of delusion is this?
(A) Somatic delusion
(B) Referential delusion
(C) Grandiose delusion
(D) Persecutory delusion

Q540. A patient begins crying uncontrollably while describing a minor inconvenience. Which emotional characteristic is this?
(A) Blunted affect
(B) Restricted affect

(C) Flat affect
(D) Labile affect

Q541. A patient frequently forgets appointments and misplaces personal items. Which cognitive function is most likely impaired?
(A) Insight
(B) Language
(C) Judgment
(D) Memory

Q542. A patient develops repetitive lip smacking and tongue movements after years of antipsychotic therapy. Which condition is present?
(A) Acute dystonia
(B) Akathisia
(C) Tardive dyskinesia
(D) Catatonia

Q543. A patient becomes convinced that everyday news broadcasts contain secret messages intended specifically for them. Which symptom is demonstrated?
(A) Delusion of reference
(B) Nihilistic delusion
(C) Somatic delusion
(D) Grandiose delusion

Q544. A patient reports feeling detached from their own body as though watching themselves from outside. Which experience is this?
(A) Depersonalization
(B) Hallucination
(C) Derealization
(D) Illusion

Q545. A patient consistently exaggerates personal achievements and expects admiration from others. Which personality trait is most evident?
(A) Dependent traits
(B) Narcissistic traits
(C) Avoidant traits
(D) Paranoid traits

Q546. A patient persistently refuses to accept the reality of a serious medical diagnosis. Which defense mechanism is this?
(A) Rationalization
(B) Denial
(C) Displacement
(D) Projection

Q547. A patient suddenly becomes mute and unresponsive while maintaining a fixed posture. Which psychiatric condition is suggested?
(A) Delirium
(B) Psychomotor agitation
(C) Akathisia
(D) Catatonia

Q548. A patient complains of persistent worry about finances, health, and family despite no immediate problems. Which disorder best explains this pattern?
(A) Specific phobia
(B) Social anxiety disorder

(C) Generalized anxiety disorder
(D) Panic disorder

Q549. A patient speaks rapidly and shifts topics quickly with superficial connections between ideas. Which thought pattern is this?
(A) Circumstantiality
(B) Tangentiality
(C) Thought blocking
(D) Flight of ideas

Q550. A patient persistently collects large quantities of objects and becomes distressed when asked to discard them. Which disorder is most consistent with this behavior?
(A) Panic disorder
(B) Obsessive-compulsive disorder
(C) Somatic symptom disorder
(D) Hoarding disorder

Q551. A patient repeatedly checks whether the door is locked even after confirming it several times. Which symptom is most clearly demonstrated?
(A) Hallucination
(B) Compulsion
(C) Delusion
(D) Illusion

Q552. A patient becomes extremely fearful and develops sweating, trembling, and palpitations within minutes of entering a crowded store. Which episode is most likely occurring?
(A) Panic attack
(B) Depressive episode
(C) Manic episode
(D) Dissociative episode

Q553. A patient insists they possess extraordinary wealth and influence despite clear evidence to the contrary. Which type of delusion is present?
(A) Nihilistic delusion
(B) Somatic delusion
(C) Grandiose delusion
(D) Persecutory delusion

Q554. A patient displays minimal emotional expression and maintains a blank facial appearance during conversation. Which affect description is most appropriate?
(A) Incongruent affect
(B) Euphoric affect
(C) Labile affect
(D) Flat affect

Q555. A patient experiences persistent fatigue, difficulty concentrating, and excessive worry for several months. Which anxiety disorder best explains these symptoms?
(A) Specific phobia
(B) Social anxiety disorder
(C) Panic disorder
(D) Generalized anxiety disorder

Q556. A patient reports seeing insects crawling on their skin despite no physical evidence. Which hallucination type is this?
(A) Visual hallucination
(B) Olfactory hallucination

(C) Tactile hallucination
(D) Auditory hallucination

Q557. A patient continues to answer questions but never directly addresses what was asked, instead giving loosely related responses. Which thought process disturbance is present?
(A) Circumstantiality
(B) Thought blocking
(C) Tangentiality
(D) Flight of ideas

Q558. A patient remains seated in a rigid posture for several hours and resists attempts to move them. Which motor symptom is present?
(A) Akathisia
(B) Dystonia
(C) Waxy flexibility
(D) Psychomotor agitation

Q559. A patient consistently attributes their personal failures to unfair treatment by others. Which defense mechanism is demonstrated?
(A) Projection
(B) Regression
(C) Identification
(D) Sublimation

Q560. A patient develops severe confusion and fluctuating levels of consciousness after a surgical procedure. Which condition is most likely present?
(A) Delirium
(B) Mania
(C) Psychosis
(D) Dementia

Q561. A patient frequently interrupts others and struggles to remain seated during conversations. Which behavioral characteristic is most evident?
(A) Social withdrawal
(B) Apathy
(C) Impulsivity
(D) Paranoia

Q562. A patient describes persistent sadness, loss of interest in hobbies, and changes in appetite lasting several weeks. Which disorder is most likely present?
(A) Schizoaffective disorder
(B) Panic disorder
(C) Major depressive disorder
(D) Bipolar disorder

Q563. A patient suddenly begins shouting and moving aggressively toward others without clear provocation. Which behavioral state is occurring?
(A) Withdrawal
(B) Catatonia
(C) Agitation
(D) Apathy

Q564. A patient repeatedly returns to the same topic despite attempts to change the conversation. Which speech pattern is this?
(A) Perseveration
(B) Neologism

(C) Circumstantiality
(D) Tangentiality

Q565. A patient believes their thoughts are being broadcast so that others can hear them. Which psychotic symptom is this?
(A) Thought insertion
(B) Delusion of control
(C) Thought broadcasting
(D) Thought withdrawal

Q566. A patient suddenly develops painful muscle contractions of the neck after receiving medication. Which adverse effect is most consistent with this presentation?
(A) Acute dystonia
(B) Parkinsonism
(C) Tardive dyskinesia
(D) Akathisia

Q567. A patient reports smelling smoke in the room even though no fire or smoke is present. Which hallucination type is this?
(A) Tactile hallucination
(B) Olfactory hallucination
(C) Visual hallucination
(D) Auditory hallucination

Q568. A patient frequently seeks reassurance from friends about minor decisions and struggles to make choices independently. Which personality pattern is suggested?
(A) Dependent traits
(B) Paranoid traits
(C) Antisocial traits
(D) Narcissistic traits

Q569. A patient laughs loudly and displays exaggerated happiness during a serious discussion about illness. Which affect description is most appropriate?
(A) Blunted affect
(B) Incongruent affect
(C) Restricted affect
(D) Flat affect

Q570. A patient persistently organizes objects in precise arrangements and becomes distressed if the order is disturbed. Which condition is most closely related to this behavior?
(A) Bipolar disorder
(B) Dissociative disorder
(C) Panic disorder
(D) Obsessive-compulsive disorder

Q571. A patient becomes convinced that their coworkers are plotting against them without evidence. Which personality trait is most consistent with this belief pattern?
(A) Paranoid traits
(B) Narcissistic traits
(C) Avoidant traits
(D) Dependent traits

Q572. A patient repeatedly engages in risky financial decisions during periods of elevated mood. Which disorder most commonly includes this behavior?
(A) Panic disorder
(B) Dissociative disorder

(C) Bipolar disorder
(D) Social anxiety disorder

Q573. A patient appears unable to recognize the seriousness of their psychiatric illness and refuses treatment. Which cognitive ability is impaired?

(A) Insight
(B) Orientation
(C) Attention
(D) Memory

Q574. A patient becomes suddenly fearful and reports that ordinary sounds seem unusually loud and threatening. Which perceptual change is this?

(A) Hallucination
(B) Hyperacusis
(C) Delusion
(D) Illusion

Q575. A patient repeatedly forgets newly learned information while long-term memories remain intact. Which memory type is primarily affected?

(A) Remote memory
(B) Short-term memory
(C) Implicit memory
(D) Procedural memory

Q576. A patient expresses intense fear that their partner will abandon them and makes frantic efforts to prevent separation. Which personality pattern may include this behavior?

(A) Obsessive traits
(B) Paranoid traits
(C) Borderline traits
(D) Schizoid traits

Q577. A patient describes feeling emotionally numb and unable to experience pleasure in previously enjoyable activities. Which symptom is present?

(A) Hyperactivity
(B) Euphoria
(C) Anhedonia
(D) Mania

Q578. A patient insists that external forces are controlling their body movements. Which delusional belief is this?

(A) Nihilistic delusion
(B) Grandiose delusion
(C) Somatic delusion
(D) Delusion of control

Q579. A patient suddenly becomes extremely restless and begins pacing rapidly around the room. Which psychomotor state is present?

(A) Psychomotor agitation
(B) Psychomotor retardation
(C) Catatonia
(D) Akinesia

Q580. A patient speaks very slowly and requires long pauses before answering questions. Which speech characteristic is observed?

(A) Poverty of speech
(B) Clang association

(C) Pressured speech
(D) Echolalia

Q581. A patient becomes anxious when separated from close family members and fears something terrible will happen to them. Which disorder is suggested?

(A) Separation anxiety disorder
(B) Specific phobia
(C) Panic disorder
(D) Social anxiety disorder

Q582. A patient repeatedly interrupts sleep due to episodes of breathing cessation. Which sleep disorder is most likely present?

(A) Sleep apnea
(B) Insomnia
(C) Parasomnia
(D) Narcolepsy

Q583. A patient suddenly loses the ability to recall personal identity after experiencing a traumatic event. Which disorder is most consistent with this presentation?

(A) Bipolar disorder
(B) Generalized anxiety disorder
(C) Panic disorder
(D) Dissociative amnesia

Q584. A patient frequently becomes irritated and angry over minor inconveniences. Which mood state is most evident?

(A) Depressed mood
(B) Irritable mood
(C) Anxious mood
(D) Euphoric mood

Q585. A patient demonstrates difficulty planning tasks and organizing daily activities. Which brain function is primarily involved?

(A) Executive functioning
(B) Motor coordination
(C) Visual perception
(D) Sensory processing

Q586. A patient persistently refuses to leave home because they believe the outside world is unsafe. Which symptom category does this belief most closely resemble?

(A) Delusion
(B) Obsession
(C) Hallucination
(D) Illusion

Q587. A patient repeatedly cleans surfaces to eliminate perceived germs even when the area appears spotless. Which behavior is demonstrated?

(A) Compulsive cleaning
(B) Dissociative behavior
(C) Avoidant behavior
(D) Phobic reaction

Q588. A patient describes persistent feelings of emptiness and unstable relationships. Which personality pattern commonly includes these experiences?

(A) Paranoid traits
(B) Schizoid traits

(C) Borderline traits
(D) Narcissistic traits

Q589. A patient becomes excessively suspicious and refuses to share personal information with healthcare providers. Which personality characteristic is most evident?

(A) Paranoid traits
(B) Narcissistic traits
(C) Avoidant traits
(D) Dependent traits

Q590. A patient suddenly experiences intense fear accompanied by chest tightness and dizziness without a clear trigger. Which condition is most likely occurring?

(A) Panic attack
(B) Dissociative episode
(C) Depressive episode
(D) Psychotic episode

Q591. A patient demonstrates repetitive blinking and shoulder shrugging that occur involuntarily. Which disorder is most consistent with these symptoms?

(A) Tic disorder
(B) Dystonia
(C) Catatonia
(D) Parkinsonism

Q592. A patient becomes increasingly withdrawn and avoids social interactions with coworkers. Which behavioral pattern is most evident?

(A) Aggression
(B) Impulsivity
(C) Social withdrawal
(D) Hyperactivity

Q593. A patient insists that they are already dead and that their body no longer exists. Which type of delusion is present?

(A) Somatic delusion
(B) Referential delusion
(C) Grandiose delusion
(D) Nihilistic delusion

Q594. A patient repeatedly avoids eye contact and appears uncomfortable during social conversations. Which emotional response is most evident?

(A) Psychosis
(B) Social anxiety
(C) Mania
(D) Catatonia

Q595. A patient demonstrates sudden uncontrolled bursts of crying and laughter. Which neurological or emotional feature is suggested?

(A) Restricted affect
(B) Emotional lability
(C) Blunted affect
(D) Flat affect

Q596. A patient persistently believes they have a severe illness despite normal medical evaluations. Which disorder is suggested?

(A) Dissociative disorder
(B) Illness anxiety disorder

(C) Panic disorder
(D) Somatic symptom disorder

Q597. A patient begins inventing new words that have meaning only to them. Which speech disturbance is this?

(A) Echolalia
(B) Neologism
(C) Perseveration
(D) Clang association

Q598. A patient refuses to move or speak for long periods despite being physically capable. Which condition is most consistent with this behavior?

(A) Delirium
(B) Psychomotor agitation
(C) Catatonia
(D) Akathisia

Q599. A patient describes intense fear of flying and refuses to travel by airplane. Which anxiety condition is most consistent with this behavior?

(A) Generalized anxiety disorder
(B) Specific phobia
(C) Social anxiety disorder
(D) Panic disorder

Q600. A patient expresses a persistent belief that strangers on the street are secretly following them. Which type of delusion is present?

(A) Grandiose delusion
(B) Somatic delusion
(C) Referential delusion
(D) Persecutory delusion

Answer Key and Explanation (501-600)

Q501. Answer: B

Explanation: This symptom refers to a marked decrease in motivation and the ability to initiate goal-directed activities. Individuals may appear apathetic and disengaged from responsibilities or social relationships. The lack of motivation can affect personal hygiene, employment, and relationships. It is categorized among the negative symptoms commonly associated with certain psychotic disorders. These symptoms often respond less robustly to treatment than positive symptoms and require long-term management strategies.

Q502. Answer: C

Explanation: This disturbance occurs when a real external stimulus is misinterpreted. The individual perceives something that exists but interprets it incorrectly due to sensory or psychological factors. Such experiences may occur in states of anxiety, fatigue, or altered consciousness. Once the actual stimulus is recognized, the misinterpretation typically resolves. Differentiating this from other perceptual disturbances is important during mental status assessment.

Q503. Answer: C

Explanation: This mood state involves elevated or irritable mood accompanied by increased activity and energy. Individuals may display grandiosity, impulsive behaviors, and reduced need for sleep. The symptoms significantly impair functioning and may require hospitalization in severe cases. The condition represents a hallmark feature of bipolar mood disorders. Accurate recognition is essential to ensure appropriate mood-stabilizing treatment.

Q504. Answer: C

Explanation: This disorder involves preoccupation with perceived physical flaws or bodily abnormalities. The concern persists even when others cannot detect any defect. Individuals often engage in repetitive behaviors such as checking mirrors or seeking reassurance. The distress can significantly interfere with social and occupational functioning. Treatment frequently includes psychotherapy aimed at modifying distorted body perceptions.

Q505. Answer: C

Explanation: Elevated levels of this neurotransmitter can lead to overstimulation within the central nervous system. Symptoms often include agitation, sweating, tremor, and changes in mental status. The reaction usually occurs when multiple medications that increase serotonin activity are combined. Early recognition is important to prevent progression to more severe complications. Treatment focuses on discontinuing the causative agents and providing supportive care.

Q506. Answer: A

Explanation: This ability allows individuals to understand concepts beyond their literal meaning. Interpreting proverbs requires reasoning about symbolic or metaphorical ideas. Difficulty with such tasks may indicate impairment in higher-level cognitive functioning. These abilities are often associated with frontal lobe activity in the brain. Assessing this skill is an important part of cognitive evaluation.

Q507. Answer: D

Explanation: This therapy involves gradual exposure to anxiety-provoking stimuli while preventing the usual compulsive response. The process helps the individual learn that anxiety will diminish without performing the ritual behavior. Over time the urge to perform the compulsive action weakens. The technique is considered a first-line behavioral treatment for obsessive behaviors. Consistent practice under therapeutic guidance improves symptom control.

Q508. Answer: D

Explanation: This condition involves intense fear of a specific object or situation. The fear is disproportionate to the actual danger posed. Individuals often avoid the triggering situation entirely. Such avoidance can interfere with normal daily activities. Behavioral therapy approaches are commonly used to gradually reduce the fear response.

Q509. Answer: B

Explanation: This belief involves the conviction that others intend to harm or sabotage the individual. The perception persists despite lack of supporting evidence. Such beliefs may lead to suspicion, mistrust, and social withdrawal. They are commonly observed in psychotic conditions. Proper evaluation helps determine the severity and guide treatment planning.

Q510. Answer: C

Explanation: This disturbance involves an abrupt interruption in the flow of thoughts. The individual may pause for several seconds and then begin speaking about an unrelated topic. It is frequently associated with psychotic disorders affecting cognitive organization. The person often reports that the thought suddenly disappeared. Recognizing this pattern helps clinicians evaluate disturbances in thinking.

Q511. Answer: B

Explanation: This symptom involves a noticeable slowing of physical and emotional reactions. Individuals may move slowly, speak less, and appear fatigued. The change reflects reduced energy and motivation commonly associated with depressive conditions. Observers may notice delays in responses or decreased spontaneous movement. Such findings help clinicians assess severity of mood disturbance.

Q512. Answer: D

Explanation: This condition involves persistent physical complaints that cause distress and disruption in daily life. Although symptoms are genuine to the individual, medical evaluations may not reveal clear physiological explanations. The individual remains preoccupied with bodily concerns. Emotional distress often accompanies the symptoms. Psychological interventions may help address underlying factors contributing to the condition.

Q513. Answer: A

Explanation: This speech pattern involves automatic repetition of words or phrases spoken by someone else. It can occur immediately after hearing the statement. The behavior is often associated with certain neurological or psychiatric conditions. Communication becomes limited because the individual does not generate independent responses. Observing such patterns can assist clinicians in diagnostic evaluation.

Q514. Answer: C

Explanation: This feature involves reduced sleep without feeling tired during the day. Individuals may remain highly active and productive despite limited rest. The change reflects heightened energy levels associated with mood elevation. Such patterns often appear early in manic episodes. Monitoring sleep patterns is important in assessing mood stability.

Q515. Answer: A

Explanation: This disorder involves intense fear of weight gain combined with severe restriction of food intake. Individuals often have distorted perceptions of body weight and shape. Despite being underweight they may believe they are overweight. The condition can lead to serious medical complications due to malnutrition. Early diagnosis and multidisciplinary treatment are essential.

Q516. Answer: C

Explanation: This disorder involves cycles of excessive food consumption followed by compensatory behaviors. Individuals often feel a loss of control during binge episodes. Purging behaviors are used to prevent weight gain. The pattern may occur secretly due to feelings of shame. Treatment commonly involves psychotherapy and nutritional counseling.

Q517. Answer: D

Explanation: This psychological process involves attributing one's own unacceptable thoughts or feelings to another person. The individual unconsciously avoids acknowledging personal responsibility. The behavior protects the ego from uncomfortable emotions such as guilt or shame. Although temporarily protective it can interfere with relationships. Recognition of such patterns can guide therapeutic discussions.

Q518. Answer: D

Explanation: This defense mechanism involves shifting emotional reactions from the original source to a safer target. The individual may feel unable to confront the true source of frustration. Instead the emotion is expressed toward someone less threatening. This process occurs unconsciously as a coping strategy. Understanding such mechanisms helps clinicians interpret behavior patterns.

Q519. Answer: C

Explanation: This observation refers to a mismatch between emotional expression and the content of speech. The person's outward emotion does not align with the seriousness of the situation described. Such discrepancies may occur in several psychiatric conditions. Observing emotional expression is an important aspect of mental status examination. Clinicians evaluate whether affect corresponds appropriately to thought content.

Q520. Answer: C

Explanation: This condition involves temporary inability to move or speak during transitions between sleep and wakefulness. The episode usually lasts only a few seconds or minutes. Individuals remain aware but unable to control voluntary muscles. It can be frightening but is generally harmless. Education and reassurance often help reduce anxiety related to these episodes.

Q521. Answer: B

Explanation: This pattern occurs when individuals assume personal responsibility for events or outcomes without evidence. They interpret neutral or positive situations as reflecting personal inadequacy. The distortion often leads to unnecessary guilt or anxiety. Such thinking patterns contribute to low self-confidence and stress. Cognitive restructuring techniques help challenge these beliefs.

Q522. Answer: C

Explanation: This domain refers to awareness of time, place, and personal identity. Difficulty identifying the current date or location indicates disorientation. Such impairment is common in various neurocognitive disorders. Orientation is typically assessed during the mental status examination. Monitoring changes in this ability helps track cognitive decline.

Q523. Answer: D

Explanation: This belief involves interpreting ordinary events as having special personal meaning. Individuals assume that unrelated actions or signals are directed specifically at them. The conviction persists even when explanations contradict the belief. Such experiences commonly occur in psychotic disorders. Recognizing these beliefs helps clinicians assess thought content abnormalities.

Q524. Answer: A

Explanation: This auditory perception involves voices giving instructions or directives. The commands may involve harmless or potentially dangerous behaviors. Such experiences are considered serious because they may influence actions. Immediate assessment of safety risk is necessary when these symptoms occur. Treatment typically involves antipsychotic medication and supportive care.

Q525. Answer: D

Explanation: This mental process allows individuals to focus on specific stimuli while ignoring irrelevant information. Impairment leads to distractibility and difficulty completing tasks. It may occur in several psychiatric or neurological conditions. Clinicians often evaluate attention using simple concentration tests. Identifying deficits helps guide further cognitive assessment.

Q526. Answer: C

Explanation: These symptoms occur when the body reacts to sudden absence of alcohol after prolonged heavy use. The nervous system becomes hyperactive due to loss of depressant effects. Early withdrawal symptoms often include tremors, anxiety, and sweating. Without treatment the condition can progress to more severe complications. Monitoring and supportive care help ensure safe recovery.

Q527. Answer: A
Explanation: This side effect involves intense inner restlessness accompanied by repetitive movements. Individuals may pace, shift weight, or be unable to sit still. The sensation can be very uncomfortable and distressing. It is commonly associated with certain medications affecting dopamine pathways. Management may involve medication adjustment or additional treatment.
Q528. Answer: B
Explanation: This phenomenon involves perception of sound in the absence of an actual auditory stimulus. Individuals may hear voices, music, or other noises. The experience is vivid and perceived as real by the person. Such symptoms often occur in psychotic or neurological conditions. Proper evaluation helps determine the underlying cause.
Q529. Answer: A
Explanation: This condition involves intense fear of situations where the individual may be judged by others. Public speaking, meeting new people, or performing in front of others often triggers anxiety. Individuals may avoid such situations to prevent embarrassment. Physical symptoms like sweating and trembling frequently occur. Effective treatment includes psychotherapy and sometimes medication.
Q530. Answer: D
Explanation: This rare but serious reaction involves severe muscle stiffness and elevated body temperature. Autonomic instability and altered consciousness may also occur. The syndrome is associated with dopamine receptor blockade from certain medications. Immediate medical intervention is required to prevent complications. Treatment typically involves stopping the medication and providing supportive care.
Q531. Answer: B
Explanation: This cognitive ability involves organizing tasks and estimating the duration needed to complete them. Impairment can lead to difficulty planning daily activities. Individuals may struggle with deadlines or punctuality. Such deficits are often associated with frontal lobe functioning. Assessing executive abilities helps determine cognitive performance.
Q532. Answer: D
Explanation: This disorder involves fear of situations where escape might be difficult or embarrassing. Individuals often avoid crowded spaces or public transportation. The avoidance behavior can severely limit independence and social activities. The fear often develops after experiencing panic attacks. Treatment typically combines psychotherapy and pharmacologic support.
Q533. Answer: C
Explanation: This speech disturbance involves linking words based on sound rather than logical meaning. Rhyming or similar sounding words may dominate the conversation. The pattern reflects disorganized thinking. It is often observed during manic episodes or psychotic states. Recognizing such speech patterns assists clinicians in evaluating thought processes.
Q534. Answer: B
Explanation: This experience involves altered perception of the external environment. Surroundings may appear dreamlike or distorted. Individuals typically recognize that the sensation is subjective rather than real. The phenomenon may occur during anxiety, trauma, or dissociative states. Proper assessment helps differentiate it from psychotic symptoms.
Q535. Answer: C
Explanation: This belief involves conviction that parts of the body or existence itself no longer function. Individuals may feel that they are dead or that their organs have ceased working. The belief persists despite medical evidence to the contrary. Such delusions can cause extreme distress. Careful psychiatric evaluation is required to determine appropriate treatment.
Q536. Answer: D

Explanation: This condition involves recurrent urges to pull out hair from the scalp, eyebrows, or other areas. The behavior often occurs in response to tension or stress. Temporary relief may follow the act of pulling. Over time the habit can lead to visible hair loss and embarrassment. Behavioral therapy is commonly used to address this repetitive behavior.

Q537. Answer: C

Explanation: This speech pattern involves a jumble of words that do not form meaningful sentences. The listener cannot follow the intended message because the language structure is disrupted. It reflects severe disorganization of thought processes. Such disturbances are often associated with acute psychosis. Recognition helps clinicians determine the severity of cognitive impairment.

Q538. Answer: C

Explanation: This condition involves intense fear directed toward a particular object or situation. The fear may be irrational but produces strong emotional and physical reactions. Individuals often avoid the feared stimulus entirely. Avoidance can interfere with daily activities or recreational interests. Behavioral exposure therapy is frequently used to reduce the fear response.

Q539. Answer: C

Explanation: This belief reflects an exaggerated sense of power or influence. Individuals may believe they possess extraordinary abilities or importance. The conviction remains fixed despite evidence that contradicts it. Such beliefs may occur in mood disorders or psychotic conditions. Proper evaluation helps determine underlying psychiatric pathology.

Q540. Answer: D

Explanation: This emotional pattern involves rapid and exaggerated changes in mood expression. Reactions may appear disproportionate to the situation. Emotional shifts can occur suddenly and unpredictably. Such findings may appear in several psychiatric or neurological conditions. Observing affect provides valuable information during mental status assessment.

Q541. Answer: D

Explanation: This mental ability allows individuals to store and retrieve information. Difficulty recalling recent events or tasks indicates impairment in memory processes. Such deficits may arise from neurological or psychiatric conditions. Memory assessment is a key component of cognitive evaluation. Early recognition helps guide diagnostic investigation.

Q542. Answer: C

Explanation: This movement disorder involves involuntary repetitive movements of the face and mouth. It typically develops after prolonged exposure to certain medications. Symptoms may persist even after discontinuation of the medication. Early detection is important to prevent progression. Regular monitoring helps identify abnormal movements during treatment.

Q543. Answer: A

Explanation: This belief involves interpreting neutral events as having personal significance. Individuals assume that messages or signals are directed specifically at them. The belief persists even when others explain alternative interpretations. Such symptoms often occur in psychotic disorders. Careful assessment helps determine appropriate treatment interventions.

Q544. Answer: A

Explanation: This phenomenon involves a sense of separation from one's physical body or mental processes. Individuals may describe feeling like an outside observer of themselves. Reality testing usually remains intact. The experience may occur during severe stress or anxiety. Clinical evaluation focuses on identifying underlying causes and triggers.

Q545. Answer: B

Explanation: This personality pattern involves an inflated sense of self-importance. Individuals often seek constant admiration and validation from others. They may exaggerate accomplishments or talents.

Interpersonal relationships may become strained due to lack of empathy. Understanding such personality features helps guide therapeutic approaches.

Q546. Answer: B

Explanation: This psychological defense involves rejecting information that causes emotional discomfort. The individual unconsciously refuses to acknowledge facts or experiences. The mechanism temporarily protects the person from distress. Over time however it may interfere with necessary medical treatment. Recognition allows clinicians to provide supportive communication.

Q547. Answer: D

Explanation: This syndrome involves disturbances in motor activity and responsiveness. Individuals may remain motionless, silent, or rigid for extended periods. The condition can occur in several psychiatric or medical disorders. Early recognition is important because specific treatments may be required. Monitoring and supportive care help prevent complications.

Q548. Answer: C

Explanation: This condition involves chronic and excessive worry about multiple life circumstances. The anxiety occurs on most days and is difficult to control. Physical symptoms such as muscle tension and fatigue are common. The constant worry interferes with concentration and sleep. Treatment usually combines psychotherapy and medication.

Q549. Answer: D

Explanation: This pattern involves accelerated thinking with rapid transitions between loosely connected ideas. Speech may be difficult to interrupt due to increased energy and excitement. The associations between ideas are often superficial. Such patterns frequently appear during manic states. Recognizing these changes helps clinicians assess mood elevation.

Q550. Answer: D

Explanation: This condition involves extreme difficulty discarding possessions regardless of their value. Items accumulate over time and clutter living spaces. Emotional attachment to objects makes removal very distressing. The behavior can impair daily functioning and create safety hazards. Psychological interventions often focus on improving decision making and organization skills.

Q551. Answer: B

Explanation: This behavior involves repetitive actions performed to relieve anxiety caused by intrusive thoughts. The individual feels driven to perform the behavior despite recognizing that it may be unnecessary. These behaviors temporarily reduce distress but reinforce the cycle of anxiety and ritualistic action. The pattern is commonly observed in obsessive-compulsive conditions. Treatment often includes behavioral interventions that focus on breaking the ritual pattern.

Q552. Answer: A

Explanation: This episode involves sudden onset of intense fear accompanied by physical symptoms. The symptoms typically peak within minutes and may include shortness of breath and chest discomfort. Individuals often feel a sense of impending danger during the event. These episodes can occur unexpectedly or be triggered by certain situations. Early recognition helps guide appropriate management and coping strategies.

Q553. Answer: C

Explanation: This belief reflects an exaggerated sense of importance or abilities. Individuals may believe they have exceptional power, knowledge, or status. The belief remains fixed even when confronted with contradictory information. Such symptoms may appear in mood disorders or psychotic conditions. Accurate identification of the belief pattern helps guide clinical treatment planning.

Q554. Answer: D

Explanation: This emotional presentation involves absence or near absence of visible emotional expression. Facial movements, tone of voice, and gestures appear limited. The individual may describe emotions internally but show little outward expression. Such patterns can occur in certain psychiatric disorders affecting emotional responsiveness. Observation of affect is a key element of mental status examination.

Q555. Answer: D

Explanation: This disorder is characterized by chronic and uncontrollable worry about multiple aspects of life. Symptoms often occur on most days for extended periods. Individuals frequently experience restlessness, fatigue, and difficulty concentrating. The anxiety interferes with normal functioning and daily activities. Treatment typically includes psychotherapy and medication when necessary.

Q556. Answer: C

Explanation: This perceptual disturbance involves the sensation of touch without a real external stimulus. Individuals may feel crawling, tingling, or movement on the skin. The experience can be distressing and may lead to scratching or skin injury. Such symptoms can occur in psychiatric or neurological conditions. Assessment focuses on identifying possible underlying causes.

Q557. Answer: C

Explanation: This thought pattern occurs when responses diverge from the original question and never return to the point. The conversation may seem loosely related but lacks a clear connection to the topic. Listeners often find it difficult to obtain direct answers. The pattern reflects impaired logical organization of thoughts. It may appear in several psychiatric conditions involving disorganized thinking.

Q558. Answer: C

Explanation: This phenomenon involves maintenance of positions imposed by another person for prolonged periods. The limbs may remain in unusual postures with minimal resistance. The behavior is often associated with catatonic states. Observing this symptom provides important clues about underlying psychiatric or neurological conditions. Prompt recognition helps guide treatment decisions.

Q559. Answer: A

Explanation: This defense mechanism involves assigning one's own undesirable feelings or thoughts to another person. The individual avoids acknowledging personal responsibility. The process operates unconsciously as a way of protecting self-esteem. Although temporarily protective, it can interfere with insight and relationships. Awareness of this pattern assists in therapeutic exploration.

Q560. Answer: A

Explanation: This condition involves sudden onset of confusion and impaired awareness. Symptoms often fluctuate throughout the day. Individuals may experience disorientation, attention deficits, and altered consciousness. Medical illness or physiological stress frequently triggers the condition. Early identification is essential because the condition is often reversible with appropriate treatment.

Q561. Answer: C

Explanation: This behavior involves acting quickly without considering consequences. Individuals may struggle with patience or waiting their turn. Impulsivity can interfere with social interactions and decision making. The trait appears in several psychiatric and developmental conditions. Recognizing the pattern helps guide behavioral interventions.

Q562. Answer: C

Explanation: This disorder involves prolonged periods of depressed mood accompanied by loss of pleasure in activities. Physical symptoms such as appetite or sleep changes frequently occur. The condition affects emotional, cognitive, and physical functioning. Symptoms must persist for a significant period to meet diagnostic criteria. Early treatment can significantly improve quality of life.

Q563. Answer: C

Explanation: This state involves excessive motor activity and emotional tension. Individuals may appear restless, irritable, or unable to remain calm. The behavior can escalate quickly if not addressed. It may occur in response to psychiatric or medical conditions. Early intervention helps ensure safety for both the patient and others.

Q564. Answer: A

Explanation: This speech disturbance involves persistent repetition of words or ideas. The individual continues focusing on the same subject even when it is no longer relevant. Such patterns may occur in neurological or psychiatric disorders. Communication may become difficult due to the repetitive nature of responses. Observing these behaviors helps guide cognitive assessment.

Q565. Answer: C

Explanation: This belief involves the conviction that private thoughts are accessible to others. Individuals may feel that their internal experiences are no longer private. The belief persists despite lack of evidence. Such symptoms often occur in certain psychotic disorders. Recognizing these experiences assists clinicians in evaluating thought content abnormalities.

Q566. Answer: A

Explanation: This reaction involves sudden sustained muscle contractions. The movements may produce abnormal postures or twisting motions. Symptoms can appear shortly after medication exposure. The condition can be distressing but often responds quickly to treatment. Prompt recognition allows rapid relief of symptoms.

Q567. Answer: B

Explanation: This perception involves detecting odors without an external stimulus. Individuals may describe smells such as smoke, chemicals, or food. The experience feels real to the person despite absence of a source. Such symptoms can occur in neurological or psychiatric conditions. Evaluation focuses on determining underlying causes.

Q568. Answer: A

Explanation: This personality pattern involves excessive reliance on others for guidance and reassurance. Individuals may feel uncomfortable making decisions alone. Fear of losing support can influence behavior and relationships. The pattern often leads to submissive or clingy behaviors. Therapeutic approaches often focus on strengthening autonomy and confidence.

Q569. Answer: B

Explanation: This emotional expression does not match the content of speech or situation. The reaction appears inappropriate to observers. Such discrepancies can provide important diagnostic information. They may occur in certain psychiatric disorders affecting emotional regulation. Evaluating affect helps clinicians understand emotional functioning.

Q570. Answer: D

Explanation: This disorder involves intrusive thoughts and repetitive behaviors performed to reduce anxiety. Individuals may feel compelled to arrange or organize items in specific ways. Disruption of the pattern can cause significant distress. The behavior often interferes with normal daily functioning. Behavioral therapy is commonly used to address these symptoms.

Q571. Answer: A

Explanation: This personality pattern involves pervasive mistrust and suspicion of others. Individuals often interpret neutral events as threatening. Relationships may become strained due to persistent doubt about others' intentions. The suspicion may occur even without clear evidence. Understanding this pattern helps clinicians plan appropriate communication strategies.

Q572. Answer: C

Explanation: This condition involves alternating periods of mood elevation and depression. During elevated mood states individuals may display impulsive behaviors such as excessive spending. Judgment may become impaired due to increased energy and confidence. These episodes can significantly affect personal and financial stability. Effective treatment focuses on mood stabilization and monitoring behavior patterns.

Q573. Answer: A

Explanation: This ability refers to awareness and understanding of one's own mental condition. Individuals with impaired insight may deny the presence of illness. Lack of awareness can interfere with treatment adherence. Clinicians often assess insight during mental status examinations. Improving understanding may enhance cooperation with care plans.

Q574. Answer: B

Explanation: This condition involves heightened sensitivity to normal environmental sounds. Everyday noises may appear excessively intense or uncomfortable. The altered perception can lead to distress or avoidance behaviors. It may occur in several neurological or psychological conditions. Assessment helps determine potential contributing factors.

Q575. Answer: B

Explanation: This memory system stores information for brief periods before it is consolidated into long-term storage. Difficulty retaining new information indicates impairment in this process. Individuals may repeat questions or forget recent conversations. Such changes often appear in early stages of cognitive disorders. Evaluating memory helps clinicians determine cognitive functioning.

Q576. Answer: C

Explanation: This personality pattern involves unstable relationships and strong fear of abandonment. Emotional responses may be intense and rapidly changing. Individuals often experience difficulty regulating emotions. Interpersonal conflicts frequently occur due to sensitivity to rejection. Therapeutic approaches focus on emotional regulation and relationship stability.

Q577. Answer: C

Explanation: This symptom refers to reduced ability to experience pleasure or satisfaction. Activities that were once enjoyable may feel meaningless. The change often accompanies depressive conditions. Loss of interest can affect motivation and daily functioning. Recognition of this symptom is important for diagnosing mood disorders.

Q578. Answer: D

Explanation: This belief involves the perception that one's actions are directed by outside forces. Individuals may feel they have lost control over their own behavior. The experience can be frightening and confusing. Such symptoms are commonly associated with certain psychotic disorders. Accurate assessment is essential for treatment planning.

Q579. Answer: A

Explanation: This condition involves increased physical activity accompanied by emotional tension. Individuals may be unable to remain still and appear highly anxious or distressed. The behavior can escalate quickly if underlying stressors remain unaddressed. It may occur in various psychiatric or medical conditions. Early intervention helps maintain safety and calm.

Q580. Answer: A

Explanation: This speech pattern involves limited verbal output and slow responses. Individuals may produce short or minimal answers. The reduced speech reflects decreased spontaneous communication. Such patterns often occur in depressive or psychotic conditions. Observing speech characteristics helps clinicians evaluate thought processes.

Q581. Answer: A

Explanation: This condition involves excessive fear related to separation from attachment figures. Individuals worry about potential harm or loss affecting loved ones. The anxiety may lead to refusal to leave home or attend activities. Symptoms can interfere with normal development and daily functioning. Treatment often includes supportive psychotherapy and coping strategies.

Q582. Answer: A

Explanation: This condition involves repeated pauses in breathing during sleep. The interruptions often cause fragmented sleep and daytime fatigue. Individuals may awaken suddenly gasping for air. The disorder can affect overall health if untreated. Evaluation typically includes sleep studies to confirm the diagnosis.

Q583. Answer: D

Explanation: This condition involves inability to recall important autobiographical information. The memory loss usually occurs after significant psychological stress or trauma. Individuals may appear confused about personal history. The condition is not due to neurological damage. Psychological support often helps recovery of memory over time.

Q584. Answer: B

Explanation: This emotional state involves increased sensitivity to frustration. Individuals may react strongly to minor stressors. The mood can fluctuate rapidly depending on circumstances. Irritability may appear in several psychiatric conditions including mood disorders. Recognizing mood patterns assists clinicians in diagnostic assessment.

Q585. Answer: A

Explanation: This cognitive domain includes skills required for planning, organizing, and decision making. It allows individuals to manage complex tasks and adapt behavior. Impairment may lead to difficulty managing responsibilities or schedules. These functions are largely associated with frontal brain regions. Assessing executive abilities helps evaluate cognitive health.

Q586. Answer: A

Explanation: This belief reflects a fixed false conviction that persists despite contrary evidence. The individual strongly believes the perceived danger is real. Such beliefs may influence behavior and limit daily functioning. They are commonly associated with certain psychiatric conditions. Careful assessment helps determine severity and underlying causes.

Q587. Answer: A

Explanation: This behavior involves repetitive actions intended to reduce anxiety about contamination. The person feels compelled to perform the cleaning ritual repeatedly. The temporary relief reinforces continuation of the behavior. Over time the ritual can consume significant time and energy. Behavioral therapy techniques are commonly used to address this pattern.

Q588. Answer: C

Explanation: This personality pattern involves intense emotional experiences and unstable interpersonal relationships. Individuals may struggle with self-image and chronic feelings of emptiness. Emotional reactions often shift rapidly in response to perceived rejection. Impulsivity and fear of abandonment are also common features. Treatment focuses on emotional regulation and interpersonal effectiveness.

Q589. Answer: A

Explanation: This pattern involves persistent mistrust of others' motives. Individuals may believe others intend to exploit or harm them. The suspicion often interferes with forming trusting relationships. Such traits may lead to reluctance in seeking or accepting help. Clinicians often need to build rapport carefully to establish trust.

Q590. Answer: A

Explanation: This episode involves sudden onset of overwhelming anxiety and physical symptoms. The sensations can be frightening and may mimic serious medical conditions. Symptoms typically peak rapidly and then gradually subside. Individuals may fear losing control or dying during the event. Education and coping strategies are essential components of management.

Q591. Answer: A

Explanation: This condition involves sudden rapid movements or vocalizations that occur repeatedly. The actions are often brief and difficult to control. Stress or excitement may increase the frequency of these behaviors. Many individuals experience temporary relief after performing the movement. Assessment helps determine severity and appropriate interventions.

Q592. Answer: C

Explanation: This behavior involves reducing or avoiding contact with others. Individuals may prefer isolation and limit participation in group activities. The change can result from anxiety, depression, or other psychological conditions. Persistent withdrawal may affect occupational and social functioning. Identifying the cause helps guide appropriate treatment strategies.

Q593. Answer: D

Explanation: This belief involves the conviction that oneself, parts of the body, or the world no longer exists. The individual may claim they are dead or empty inside. The belief persists despite clear contradictory evidence. Such symptoms are rare but can appear in severe psychiatric conditions. Immediate psychiatric evaluation is necessary to ensure safety and treatment.

Q594. Answer: B

Explanation: This response involves fear of negative evaluation in social situations. Individuals may feel embarrassed or self-conscious when interacting with others. Physical symptoms such as sweating or trembling can accompany the anxiety. Avoidance of conversations or eye contact is common. Treatment often includes cognitive and behavioral interventions.

Q595. Answer: B

Explanation: This pattern involves rapid and exaggerated changes in emotional expression. The emotional reactions may appear disproportionate to the situation. Such fluctuations can occur due to neurological or psychiatric conditions. Observers may find the responses unpredictable. Assessment helps determine underlying causes affecting emotional regulation.

Q596. Answer: B

Explanation: This condition involves preoccupation with having or acquiring a serious illness. The individual interprets normal bodily sensations as signs of disease. Reassurance from medical professionals rarely reduces the worry. Anxiety about health becomes the central focus of concern. Psychological therapy often helps address the persistent fear.

Q597. Answer: B

Explanation: This speech pattern involves creation of new words or phrases not recognized by others. The invented terms often carry specific meaning to the individual. Such patterns reflect disorganized language processing. They may occur in certain psychotic disorders. Recognizing unusual speech patterns assists clinicians in assessing thought disturbances.

Q598. Answer: C

Explanation: This syndrome involves marked disturbances in motor behavior and responsiveness. Individuals may remain motionless or silent for extended periods. The condition can occur in association with several psychiatric disorders. Early recognition is important because specific treatments may improve symptoms. Monitoring physical health is also essential during episodes.

Q599. Answer: B

Explanation: This condition involves strong fear related to a particular object or situation. The fear is excessive compared with the actual risk involved. Individuals often avoid the situation entirely to prevent anxiety. Avoidance can interfere with travel, work, or leisure activities. Behavioral exposure therapy is frequently used to reduce the fear response.

Q600. Answer: D

Explanation: This belief involves the conviction that others intend to harm or monitor the individual. The suspicion persists even when there is no evidence to support it. Such beliefs may lead to heightened fear and avoidance of others. They are commonly associated with psychotic disorders. Careful evaluation helps determine appropriate treatment and support.

Question (601-700)

Q601. A psychiatric nurse practitioner evaluates a patient who reports hearing voices that comment on their actions throughout the day. The patient states the voices often narrate what they are doing, such as when eating or walking. Which symptom is most consistent with this description?

(A) Thought broadcasting
(B) Thought insertion
(C) Illusion
(D) Auditory hallucination

Q602. A patient with major depressive disorder reports persistent fatigue, decreased concentration, and loss of interest in previously enjoyable activities for several months. Which neurochemical change is most associated with these symptoms?

(A) Increased acetylcholine
(B) Decreased serotonin
(C) Increased norepinephrine
(D) Increased dopamine

Q603. A patient with bipolar disorder presents with increased energy, decreased need for sleep, rapid speech, and impulsive spending behaviors lasting several days. Which mood episode is most consistent with these findings?

(A) Dysthymic episode
(B) Hypomanic episode
(C) Cyclothymic episode
(D) Major depressive episode

Q604. A patient admitted to a psychiatric unit repeatedly states that their internal organs have stopped functioning even though medical tests are normal. Which type of delusion is most consistent with this belief?

(A) Persecutory
(B) Nihilistic
(C) Grandiose
(D) Somatic

Q605. During an interview, a patient abruptly changes topics with only loose connections between ideas, making the conversation difficult to follow. Which thought process disturbance best describes this pattern?

(A) Loose associations
(B) Flight of ideas
(C) Circumstantiality
(D) Tangentiality

Q606. A patient taking an antipsychotic medication develops muscle rigidity, tremors, and slowed movements several weeks after starting treatment. Which adverse effect is most likely occurring?

(A) Tardive dyskinesia
(B) Parkinsonism
(C) Neuroleptic malignant syndrome
(D) Akathisia

Q607. A patient hospitalized for alcohol withdrawal begins experiencing visual hallucinations, severe agitation, fever, and fluctuating levels of consciousness two days after the last drink. Which condition is most consistent with these findings?

(A) Alcohol intoxication
(B) Wernicke encephalopathy

(C) Korsakoff syndrome
(D) Delirium tremens

Q608. A patient repeatedly washes their hands dozens of times daily due to fear of contamination despite recognizing the behavior is excessive. Which disorder is most consistent with this presentation?
(A) Generalized anxiety disorder
(B) Panic disorder
(C) Social anxiety disorder
(D) Obsessive-compulsive disorder

Q609. A patient states that coworkers are secretly plotting to harm them and insists that the organization is monitoring all of their actions. Which symptom category best describes this belief?
(A) Referential delusion
(B) Persecutory delusion
(C) Grandiose delusion
(D) Somatic delusion

Q610. A patient experiencing severe anxiety reports sudden episodes of intense fear accompanied by chest pain, dizziness, and a feeling of impending doom that peaks within minutes. Which condition is most consistent with these symptoms?
(A) Specific phobia
(B) Adjustment disorder
(C) Acute stress disorder
(D) Panic attack

Q611. A patient with schizophrenia demonstrates minimal facial expression, reduced speech, and lack of motivation for daily activities. Which type of symptom is being observed?
(A) Mood symptom
(B) Cognitive symptom
(C) Negative symptom
(D) Positive symptom

Q612. A patient reports persistent worry about multiple areas of life including finances, health, and family responsibilities for more than six months. The worry is difficult to control and accompanied by restlessness and muscle tension. Which disorder is most consistent with this presentation?
(A) Social anxiety disorder
(B) Generalized anxiety disorder
(C) Acute stress disorder
(D) Panic disorder

Q613. A patient reports recurrent intrusive memories and nightmares following a traumatic event that occurred several months earlier. The patient also avoids reminders of the event and experiences heightened startle responses. Which disorder is most consistent with these symptoms?
(A) Adjustment disorder
(B) Panic disorder
(C) Acute stress disorder
(D) Post-traumatic stress disorder

Q614. A patient begins pacing constantly and reports feeling extremely restless shortly after starting an antipsychotic medication. Which medication side effect is most consistent with these symptoms?
(A) Akathisia
(B) Tardive dyskinesia
(C) Dystonia
(D) Parkinsonism

Q615. A patient demonstrates repetitive lip smacking and involuntary tongue movements after taking antipsychotic medication for several years. Which condition is most likely responsible?
(A) Tardive dyskinesia
(B) Neuroleptic malignant syndrome
(C) Serotonin syndrome
(D) Acute dystonia
Q616. A patient hospitalized for depression expresses feelings of worthlessness and states that life has no meaning. Which psychological concept is most closely related to this experience?
(A) Anhedonia
(B) Delusion
(C) Hopelessness
(D) Dissociation
Q617. A patient undergoing a mental status examination is unable to recall three words after five minutes. Which cognitive function is being evaluated?
(A) Abstract reasoning
(B) Immediate memory
(C) Remote memory
(D) Recent memory
Q618. A patient reports persistent sadness but continues to function at work and maintain relationships. The symptoms have lasted for more than two years. Which disorder is most consistent with this presentation?
(A) Persistent depressive disorder
(B) Major depressive disorder
(C) Bipolar disorder
(D) Adjustment disorder
Q619. A patient suddenly develops severe muscle stiffness, high fever, confusion, and unstable blood pressure after starting an antipsychotic medication. Which condition should be suspected?
(A) Akathisia
(B) Acute dystonia
(C) Neuroleptic malignant syndrome
(D) Serotonin syndrome
Q620. A patient describes a persistent fear of being in crowded places because escape may be difficult if anxiety develops. Which condition best describes this fear?
(A) Agoraphobia
(B) Panic disorder
(C) Social anxiety disorder
(D) Specific phobia
Q621. A patient believes that news anchors on television are sending them secret messages meant specifically for them. Which type of delusion is most consistent with this belief?
(A) Grandiose delusion
(B) Nihilistic delusion
(C) Referential delusion
(D) Somatic delusion
Q622. During a psychiatric interview, a patient provides excessive and unnecessary details before eventually answering the original question. Which thought process pattern is most consistent with this behavior?
(A) Blocking
(B) Flight of ideas

(C) Circumstantiality
(D) Tangentiality

Q623. A patient abruptly stops speaking in the middle of a sentence and cannot recall what they were saying moments earlier. Which thought disturbance best describes this phenomenon?

(A) Tangential thinking
(B) Echolalia
(C) Thought insertion
(D) Thought blocking

Q624. A patient reports feeling detached from their own body and describes the sensation as if they are observing themselves from outside their body. Which experience best describes this symptom?

(A) Depersonalization
(B) Dissociation
(C) Delusion
(D) Derealization

Q625. A patient believes they possess extraordinary powers and insists they have a special mission to save the world. Which type of delusion is most consistent with this belief?

(A) Grandiose
(B) Somatic
(C) Persecutory
(D) Referential

Q626. A patient taking selective serotonin reuptake inhibitors develops agitation, sweating, tremors, and confusion after combining the medication with another serotonergic drug. Which condition should be suspected?

(A) Tardive dyskinesia
(B) Neuroleptic malignant syndrome
(C) Acute dystonia
(D) Serotonin syndrome

Q627. A patient states that they feel emotionally numb and unable to experience pleasure from activities that were previously enjoyable. Which symptom is most consistent with this description?

(A) Catatonia
(B) Mania
(C) Apathy
(D) Anhedonia

Q628. A patient repeatedly mimics the words spoken by the interviewer during a psychiatric assessment. Which term best describes this behavior?

(A) Perseveration
(B) Echopraxia
(C) Neologism
(D) Echolalia

Q629. A patient appears immobile, maintains a fixed posture for extended periods, and shows minimal response to external stimuli. Which condition best describes this presentation?

(A) Catatonia
(B) Anxiety disorder
(C) Delirium
(D) Mania

Q630. A patient demonstrates rapid speech, distractibility, and continuous shifting between topics during an interview. Which thought pattern is most consistent with these observations?

(A) Flight of ideas

(B) Tangential thinking
(C) Thought blocking
(D) Circumstantial thinking

Q631. A patient experiences persistent fear of social situations due to concerns about being judged or embarrassed by others. Which condition is most consistent with this presentation?
(A) Agoraphobia
(B) Panic disorder
(C) Generalized anxiety disorder
(D) Social anxiety disorder

Q632. A patient reports repeatedly checking that doors are locked before leaving home, sometimes returning multiple times to confirm. Which psychological mechanism is most closely related to this behavior?
(A) Delusion
(B) Phobia
(C) Compulsion
(D) Dissociation

Q633. A patient presents with fluctuating levels of consciousness, disorientation, and difficulty maintaining attention over several hours. Which condition is most consistent with these findings?
(A) Delirium
(B) Schizophrenia
(C) Depression
(D) Dementia

Q634. A patient expresses persistent feelings of emptiness and unstable relationships characterized by alternating idealization and intense anger. Which personality disorder is most consistent with this pattern?
(A) Borderline personality disorder
(B) Avoidant personality disorder
(C) Narcissistic personality disorder
(D) Antisocial personality disorder

Q635. A patient reports persistent difficulty falling asleep despite feeling tired and spending sufficient time in bed each night. Which sleep disorder is most consistent with this complaint?
(A) Narcolepsy
(B) Insomnia disorder
(C) Sleep apnea
(D) Parasomnia

Q636. A patient repeatedly pulls out their hair resulting in noticeable hair loss. Which disorder is most consistent with this behavior?
(A) Illness anxiety disorder
(B) Somatic symptom disorder
(C) Body dysmorphic disorder
(D) Trichotillomania

Q637. A patient insists they are infested with insects crawling under their skin despite medical evidence showing no infestation. Which type of delusion is most consistent with this belief?
(A) Grandiose delusion
(B) Somatic delusion
(C) Persecutory delusion
(D) Referential delusion

Q638. A patient frequently invents new words that have meaning only to them during conversation. Which term best describes this behavior?
(A) Clang association
(B) Perseveration
(C) Echolalia
(D) Neologism
Q639. A patient with depression reports waking several hours earlier than usual and being unable to return to sleep. Which sleep pattern disturbance is most consistent with this complaint?
(A) Hypersomnia
(B) Early morning awakening
(C) Sleep paralysis
(D) Sleepwalking
Q640. A patient demonstrates persistent disregard for the rights of others and repeatedly engages in deceptive and manipulative behaviors. Which personality disorder is most consistent with this pattern?
(A) Narcissistic personality disorder
(B) Obsessive-compulsive personality disorder
(C) Dependent personality disorder
(D) Antisocial personality disorder
Q641. A patient frequently interrupts others, struggles to remain seated during meetings, and reports difficulty completing tasks due to constant distraction. Which disorder is most consistent with these symptoms?
(A) Conduct disorder
(B) Attention-deficit/hyperactivity disorder
(C) Generalized anxiety disorder
(D) Bipolar disorder
Q642. A patient reports sudden episodes of falling asleep during daytime activities such as conversations or meals despite adequate nighttime sleep. Which sleep disorder is most consistent with this presentation?
(A) Restless legs syndrome
(B) Narcolepsy
(C) Sleep apnea
(D) Insomnia disorder
Q643. A patient experiencing severe stress begins forgetting important personal information and cannot recall events from the past several hours. Which condition best describes this memory disturbance?
(A) Dissociative amnesia
(B) Delirium
(C) Dementia
(D) Schizophrenia
Q644. A patient repeatedly expresses fear of developing serious illness despite medical evaluations showing no evidence of disease. Which disorder is most consistent with this behavior?
(A) Somatic symptom disorder
(B) Body dysmorphic disorder
(C) Conversion disorder
(D) Illness anxiety disorder
Q645. A patient becomes extremely anxious when confronted with a specific object such as spiders and avoids environments where the object may be present. Which disorder best describes this pattern?
(A) Agoraphobia

(B) Panic disorder
(C) Specific phobia
(D) Social anxiety disorder

Q646. A patient reports persistent feelings of detachment from the surrounding environment and describes the world as unreal or dreamlike. Which experience best describes this symptom?
(A) Depersonalization
(B) Delusion
(C) Derealization
(D) Dissociation

Q647. A patient persistently repeats the same word or phrase in response to different questions during an interview. Which speech disturbance best describes this pattern?
(A) Neologism
(B) Perseveration
(C) Echolalia
(D) Clang association

Q648. A patient reports experiencing recurrent urges to steal items that are not needed or valuable and feels relief after taking them. Which disorder is most consistent with this behavior?
(A) Kleptomania
(B) Conduct disorder
(C) Antisocial personality disorder
(D) Obsessive-compulsive disorder

Q649. A patient begins displaying excessive energy, decreased need for sleep, inflated self-esteem, and engaging in risky activities for more than a week. Which episode is most consistent with these findings?
(A) Manic episode
(B) Hypomanic episode
(C) Mixed episode
(D) Depressive episode

Q650. A patient experiences sudden weakness in one arm after a stressful event, yet neurological examinations show no physical cause. Which condition is most consistent with this presentation?
(A) Malingering
(B) Conversion disorder
(C) Somatic symptom disorder
(D) Factitious disorder

Q651. A patient states that their thoughts are being broadcast aloud so that others can hear them. Which type of delusion is most consistent with this belief?
(A) Grandiose delusion
(B) Thought broadcasting
(C) Referential delusion
(D) Persecutory delusion

Q652. A patient suddenly loses the ability to speak following a traumatic event but shows no neurological damage. Which disorder best explains this symptom?
(A) Conversion disorder
(B) Somatic symptom disorder
(C) Factitious disorder
(D) Dissociative identity disorder

Q653. A patient repeatedly checks their appearance in mirrors due to intense concern about a perceived flaw in their appearance. Which disorder is most consistent with this behavior?
(A) Somatic symptom disorder

(B) Illness anxiety disorder
(C) Delusional disorder
(D) Body dysmorphic disorder

Q654. A patient suddenly begins speaking rapidly with rhyming words that sound similar but lack meaningful connection. Which speech pattern best describes this behavior?
(A) Echolalia
(B) Clang association
(C) Perseveration
(D) Neologism

Q655. A patient expresses intense fear of abandonment and engages in impulsive behaviors during emotional distress. Which personality disorder is most consistent with this pattern?
(A) Narcissistic personality disorder
(B) Avoidant personality disorder
(C) Borderline personality disorder
(D) Dependent personality disorder

Q656. A patient shows persistent inability to maintain attention during a mental status examination and becomes easily distracted by background noises. Which cognitive function is primarily impaired?
(A) Judgment
(B) Attention
(C) Orientation
(D) Insight

Q657. A patient becomes extremely anxious when separated from a close family member and fears that harm will occur if they are apart. Which disorder is most consistent with this pattern?
(A) Panic disorder
(B) Separation anxiety disorder
(C) Agoraphobia
(D) Social anxiety disorder

Q658. A patient repeatedly organizes objects in symmetrical patterns and becomes distressed if the arrangement is disrupted. Which disorder is most consistent with this behavior?
(A) Obsessive-compulsive personality disorder
(B) Obsessive-compulsive disorder
(C) Specific phobia
(D) Generalized anxiety disorder

Q659. A patient experiences vivid hallucinations shortly after waking from sleep and feels temporarily unable to move. Which sleep-related phenomenon best explains this experience?
(A) Narcolepsy
(B) Sleepwalking
(C) Night terrors
(D) Sleep paralysis

Q660. A patient demonstrates sudden, repetitive movements such as blinking and shoulder shrugging that occur involuntarily. Which disorder is most consistent with these symptoms?
(A) Somatic symptom disorder
(B) Tourette disorder
(C) Panic disorder
(D) Conversion disorder

Q661. A patient believes that strangers passing by on the street are actually secret agents assigned to follow them. Which type of delusion best describes this belief?
(A) Referential delusion

(B) Persecutory delusion
(C) Somatic delusion
(D) Grandiose delusion

Q662. A patient repeatedly washes their clothes multiple times because they feel the items are contaminated even after cleaning. Which psychological phenomenon is most closely related to this behavior?
(A) Obsession
(B) Delusion
(C) Phobia
(D) Compulsion

Q663. A patient describes feeling extremely energetic, sleeping only a few hours per night, and starting multiple ambitious projects simultaneously. Which mood disturbance is most consistent with this description?
(A) Depression
(B) Mania
(C) Anxiety
(D) Dysthymia

Q664. A patient undergoing a mental status exam correctly identifies the current year and location but cannot explain similarities between objects such as an apple and an orange. Which cognitive ability is impaired?
(A) Orientation
(B) Abstract reasoning
(C) Memory
(D) Attention

Q665. A patient persistently exaggerates physical symptoms and frequently seeks medical attention despite normal test results. Which disorder is most consistent with this pattern?
(A) Conversion disorder
(B) Delusional disorder
(C) Illness anxiety disorder
(D) Somatic symptom disorder

Q666. A patient becomes extremely anxious when required to speak in front of a group and avoids presentations whenever possible. Which disorder is most consistent with this presentation?
(A) Panic disorder
(B) Agoraphobia
(C) Social anxiety disorder
(D) Specific phobia

Q667. A patient hospitalized for psychiatric care suddenly begins maintaining rigid body positions for long periods and resists attempts to move them. Which condition best describes this behavior?
(A) Mania
(B) Catatonia
(C) Dissociation
(D) Delirium

Q668. A patient suddenly experiences an overwhelming fear accompanied by rapid heartbeat, sweating, and shortness of breath without any clear external trigger. Which condition best explains this episode?
(A) Specific phobia
(B) Adjustment disorder
(C) Generalized anxiety disorder

(D) Panic attack

Q669. A patient frequently exaggerates achievements and expects special treatment due to a belief of superior importance. Which personality disorder is most consistent with this pattern?

(A) Avoidant personality disorder
(B) Narcissistic personality disorder
(C) Borderline personality disorder
(D) Dependent personality disorder

Q670. A patient reports sudden weakness in both legs after experiencing severe emotional distress, yet neurological tests reveal no abnormalities. Which diagnosis is most consistent with this presentation?

(A) Factitious disorder
(B) Conversion disorder
(C) Somatic symptom disorder
(D) Malingering

Q671. A patient repeatedly organizes books and objects in perfect alignment and becomes distressed when the arrangement is disturbed. Which disorder is most consistent with this behavior?

(A) Specific phobia
(B) Obsessive-compulsive personality disorder
(C) Obsessive-compulsive disorder
(D) Generalized anxiety disorder

Q672. A patient reports hearing voices discussing their actions even when no one else is present. Which perceptual disturbance best describes this symptom?

(A) Derealization
(B) Illusion
(C) Delusion
(D) Auditory hallucination

Q673. A patient repeatedly steals small items from stores despite having no financial need and later feels guilt about the behavior. Which disorder is most consistent with this pattern?

(A) Antisocial personality disorder
(B) Kleptomania
(C) Obsessive-compulsive disorder
(D) Conduct disorder

Q674. A patient during a mental status exam cannot identify the current date or location but recognizes familiar people. Which cognitive domain is primarily impaired?

(A) Orientation
(B) Attention
(C) Insight
(D) Memory

Q675. A patient believes their body is emitting a foul odor that others can smell even though no odor is present. Which type of delusion best describes this belief?

(A) Grandiose delusion
(B) Persecutory delusion
(C) Referential delusion
(D) Somatic delusion

Q676. A patient appears extremely fatigued during the day due to repeated interruptions in breathing during sleep. Which sleep disorder is most consistent with this description?

(A) Sleep apnea
(B) Sleepwalking
(C) Insomnia disorder

(D) Narcolepsy

Q677. A patient suddenly becomes confused and disoriented while hospitalized for an infection and has difficulty maintaining attention. Which condition is most consistent with these findings?

(A) Schizophrenia
(B) Dementia
(C) Depression
(D) Delirium

Q678. A patient feels compelled to repeat certain numbers while counting objects because failing to do so causes intense anxiety. Which psychological concept best explains this behavior?

(A) Delusion
(B) Hallucination
(C) Compulsion
(D) Dissociation

Q679. A patient experiences intense sadness, fatigue, and loss of interest in activities nearly every day for several weeks. Which disorder is most consistent with these symptoms?

(A) Cyclothymic disorder
(B) Bipolar disorder
(C) Major depressive disorder
(D) Persistent depressive disorder

Q680. A patient persistently depends on others to make everyday decisions and fears being alone. Which personality disorder is most consistent with this pattern?

(A) Dependent personality disorder
(B) Narcissistic personality disorder
(C) Avoidant personality disorder
(D) Antisocial personality disorder

Q681. A patient repeatedly pulls out their hair when feeling stressed, leading to noticeable hair loss. Which disorder best describes this behavior?

(A) Trichotillomania
(B) Conversion disorder
(C) Body dysmorphic disorder
(D) Excoriation disorder

Q682. A patient insists that a television news anchor is sending them secret messages through hand gestures during broadcasts. Which type of delusion does this represent?

(A) Grandiose delusion
(B) Referential delusion
(C) Nihilistic delusion
(D) Somatic delusion

Q683. A patient with severe depression reports feeling as though their body organs have stopped functioning and that they are already dead. Which type of delusion is this?

(A) Somatic delusion
(B) Referential delusion
(C) Grandiose delusion
(D) Nihilistic delusion

Q684. A patient suddenly leaves home and travels to another city without remembering their identity or past life. Which disorder best describes this condition?

(A) Depersonalization disorder
(B) Dissociative identity disorder
(C) Dissociative amnesia with fugue

(D) Acute stress disorder

Q685. A patient feels detached from their own body and describes the sensation as observing themselves from outside. Which experience is this?

(A) Dissociation

(B) Derealization

(C) Hallucination

(D) Depersonalization

Q686. A patient persistently worries about everyday situations such as finances, work, and health for more than six months. Which disorder is most consistent with this pattern?

(A) Social anxiety disorder

(B) Generalized anxiety disorder

(C) Specific phobia

(D) Panic disorder

Q687. A patient reports sleeping only two hours per night yet feeling extremely energetic and productive. Which symptom of mania does this demonstrate?

(A) Circadian rhythm disturbance

(B) Reduced need for sleep

(C) Insomnia

(D) Sleep deprivation disorder

Q688. A patient repeatedly checks that the door is locked dozens of times before leaving the house. Which symptom is this an example of?

(A) Delusion

(B) Compulsion

(C) Obsession

(D) Hallucination

Q689. A patient believes they possess extraordinary powers and a special mission to save humanity. Which type of delusion is this?

(A) Referential delusion

(B) Persecutory delusion

(C) Somatic delusion

(D) Grandiose delusion

Q690. A patient reports seeing insects crawling on the walls when none are present. Which perceptual disturbance is this?

(A) Depersonalization

(B) Illusion

(C) Delusion

(D) Hallucination

Q691. A patient becomes extremely frightened when entering elevators and avoids them whenever possible. Which condition best explains this fear?

(A) Panic disorder

(B) Social anxiety disorder

(C) Agoraphobia

(D) Specific phobia

Q692. A patient has difficulty remembering recent conversations but recalls events from childhood clearly. Which type of memory impairment is suggested?

(A) Procedural memory loss

(B) Long-term memory impairment

(C) Short-term memory impairment

(D) Sensory memory loss

Q693. A patient frequently engages in reckless behaviors and disregards the rights of others without remorse. Which personality disorder is most consistent with this pattern?

(A) Narcissistic personality disorder
(B) Borderline personality disorder
(C) Antisocial personality disorder
(D) Dependent personality disorder

Q694. A patient who experienced a traumatic accident has repeated flashbacks and nightmares about the event. Which disorder is most likely?

(A) Post-traumatic stress disorder
(B) Panic disorder
(C) Adjustment disorder
(D) Acute stress disorder

Q695. A patient consistently interprets neutral facial expressions of others as hostile or threatening. Which cognitive distortion does this represent?

(A) Misinterpretation of social cues
(B) Projection
(C) Thought blocking
(D) Delusional thinking

Q696. A patient complains of persistent fatigue and difficulty concentrating after long-term stress at work. Which condition may best explain these symptoms?

(A) Burnout syndrome
(B) Panic disorder
(C) Bipolar disorder
(D) Psychotic disorder

Q697. A patient states that their thoughts are being controlled by an external force. Which psychotic symptom does this represent?

(A) Thought control delusion
(B) Thought broadcasting
(C) Thought insertion
(D) Thought blocking

Q698. A patient abruptly stops speaking in the middle of a sentence and cannot recall what they were saying. Which thought process disturbance is this?

(A) Thought blocking
(B) Tangential thinking
(C) Flight of ideas
(D) Circumstantial thinking

Q699. A patient displays rapid speech, jumping quickly from one topic to another with loosely connected ideas. Which thought pattern does this indicate?

(A) Flight of ideas
(B) Circumstantial thinking
(C) Thought blocking
(D) Tangential thinking

Q700. During a mental status examination, a patient denies having any mental health problems despite clear symptoms affecting daily functioning. Which concept best describes this response?

(A) Judgment
(B) Lack of insight
(C) Orientation impairment

(D) Insight

Answer Key and Explanation (601-700)

Q601. Answer: D

Explanation: Hearing voices without an external auditory stimulus represents a perceptual experience generated internally by the brain. This phenomenon occurs when the sensory system processes signals that are not actually present in the environment. The experience often feels very real to the person and may involve voices speaking directly or commenting on actions. Such symptoms are frequently associated with psychotic disorders and may cause significant distress or distraction. The perception is not caused by misinterpretation of real sounds but by internally produced sensory activity. Clinical evaluation focuses on identifying underlying psychiatric conditions. Treatment usually involves antipsychotic medications and supportive therapy.

Q602. Answer: B

Explanation: Mood regulation in the brain is strongly influenced by several neurotransmitters that coordinate emotional balance. Serotonin plays a key role in regulating mood, sleep patterns, appetite, and emotional stability. When serotonin levels decrease, individuals may experience persistent sadness, low energy, and diminished interest in daily activities. This imbalance can also affect concentration and motivation. Neurochemical dysregulation is a central factor in many depressive disorders. Modern antidepressant therapies frequently work by increasing serotonin availability in neural pathways. Improvement in mood often occurs gradually as neurotransmitter balance is restored.

Q603. Answer: B

Explanation: Elevated mood combined with increased energy and reduced need for sleep indicates an abnormal state of heightened activity. Individuals may feel unusually confident, talkative, and productive during this period. Behavioral impulsivity, such as excessive spending or risk-taking, is also common. Despite the increased energy, the disturbance may not cause severe functional impairment. These episodes represent a milder form of mania and are characteristic of certain bipolar conditions. The mood elevation may appear positive initially but can still lead to poor judgment. Early recognition allows clinicians to adjust mood stabilizing treatment appropriately.

Q604. Answer: B

Explanation: This belief reflects a fixed false idea involving themes of nonexistence or extreme bodily deterioration. Individuals may believe that parts of their body are missing, destroyed, or no longer functioning. The conviction remains strong even when objective evidence shows normal functioning. Such beliefs often appear in severe mood or psychotic conditions. The person may experience profound hopelessness and emotional distress. These ideas are not simply health concerns but deeply held distorted beliefs. Treatment focuses on addressing the underlying psychiatric disorder through medication and therapy.

Q605. Answer: A

Explanation: This thinking pattern occurs when ideas shift rapidly without a clear logical relationship. The person may jump from one topic to another with minimal connection between statements. As a result, communication becomes confusing and difficult to follow. The disturbance reflects disorganized thought processes rather than intentional behavior. It is often observed in certain psychotic disorders where cognitive organization is impaired. Listeners may struggle to identify how the conversation progressed between ideas. Careful clinical assessment helps determine the severity of the underlying condition. Treatment typically targets the psychiatric disorder affecting thought organization.

Q606. Answer: B

Explanation: These motor symptoms resemble the movement abnormalities seen in Parkinson's disease. They occur because certain medications block dopamine receptors in pathways responsible for movement control. As dopamine activity decreases, muscle stiffness, tremor, and slowed movement may develop. Facial expression may become reduced and gait may appear shuffling. These symptoms usually emerge within weeks of initiating treatment. Monitoring neurological signs is important when prescribing medications affecting dopamine pathways. Early detection allows clinicians to adjust therapy or add medications that reduce these side effects. Effective management improves patient comfort and adherence to treatment.

Q607. Answer: D

Explanation: This severe withdrawal condition occurs when chronic heavy alcohol consumption suddenly stops. The nervous system becomes hyperactive because it had previously adapted to the depressant effects of alcohol. Symptoms include confusion, hallucinations, agitation, and marked autonomic instability. Physiological signs such as fever, elevated heart rate, and blood pressure are common. The individual's level of consciousness may fluctuate rapidly. Without prompt medical treatment, the condition can become life-threatening. Management requires close monitoring and medications that stabilize the nervous system. Early recognition significantly reduces the risk of complications.

Q608. Answer: D

Explanation: This condition involves intrusive thoughts that create intense anxiety or discomfort. The person attempts to relieve this distress through repetitive behaviors or rituals. These behaviors may temporarily reduce anxiety but reinforce the cycle over time. Individuals often recognize that the behavior is excessive yet feel unable to stop it. The rituals can become time-consuming and interfere with normal daily functioning. The disorder involves both persistent thoughts and repetitive actions aimed at reducing distress. Treatment commonly includes cognitive behavioral therapy and medications affecting serotonin pathways.

Q609. Answer: B

Explanation: This belief involves the conviction that others intend to cause harm or are actively targeting the individual. The person interprets neutral or unrelated events as evidence of a threatening conspiracy. These ideas persist even when there is no objective proof supporting them. Such beliefs often produce intense fear, distrust, or defensive behavior. Logical explanations rarely change the individual's conviction. These symptoms are frequently associated with psychotic disorders. Clinical treatment focuses on reducing the severity of distorted beliefs and improving insight.

Q610. Answer: D

Explanation: This experience involves a sudden surge of intense fear that reaches peak intensity within a short period. Physical symptoms commonly include chest discomfort, rapid heartbeat, dizziness, and shortness of breath. Individuals often feel as if something catastrophic is about to happen. The episode may occur unexpectedly and without a clear external trigger. Although the symptoms can feel life-threatening, they usually resolve within minutes. Repeated episodes may cause individuals to worry about having additional attacks. Treatment often includes psychotherapy and medications that help regulate anxiety responses.

Q611. Answer: C

Explanation: These manifestations represent reductions in normal emotional and behavioral functioning. Individuals may show limited facial expression, diminished speech output, and decreased motivation. Social withdrawal and reduced emotional responsiveness are also common. These symptoms reflect a loss or absence of typical psychological functions. They tend to persist longer than acute psychotic symptoms and may significantly impair daily functioning. The condition often affects the ability to maintain relationships or employment. Treatment includes antipsychotic medication and psychosocial rehabilitation strategies.

Q612. Answer: B

Explanation: This disorder involves excessive and persistent worry about a wide range of everyday situations. The anxiety occurs more days than not and is difficult for the individual to control. Physical symptoms often accompany the worry, including muscle tension, fatigue, and restlessness. Concentration difficulties and sleep disturbances are also common. The persistent anxiety interferes with normal daily functioning. Unlike episodic panic symptoms, the worry is continuous rather than sudden. Treatment often combines psychotherapy and medications that reduce chronic anxiety.

Q613. Answer: D

Explanation: This disorder develops after exposure to a traumatic experience involving threat or serious harm. Individuals may repeatedly relive the event through distressing memories or nightmares. Avoidance of reminders related to the trauma is common. Emotional numbness and heightened alertness may also occur. The symptoms persist for an extended period and significantly disrupt daily life. Increased startle responses and sleep disturbances are frequently reported. Treatment often includes trauma-focused psychotherapy and supportive interventions.

Q614. Answer: A

Explanation: This condition involves an intense internal feeling of restlessness combined with an inability to remain still. Individuals may pace, shift weight frequently, or feel compelled to keep moving. The discomfort can become extremely distressing and may worsen adherence to medication. It often appears soon after initiation or dose increase of certain medications. The symptoms are related to dopamine receptor blockade affecting motor control pathways. Early recognition allows clinicians to adjust medication therapy. Management may include dose changes or medications that reduce restlessness.

Q615. Answer: A

Explanation: This movement disorder develops after prolonged exposure to medications affecting dopamine pathways. It involves repetitive, involuntary movements often affecting the mouth, tongue, or face. The symptoms may gradually worsen over time if the medication continues. The underlying mechanism involves long-term changes in dopamine receptor sensitivity. Because the condition may become irreversible, early detection is critical. Clinicians often monitor patients regularly for abnormal movements. Treatment may involve adjusting medication or using agents designed to reduce abnormal motor activity.

Q616. Answer: C

Explanation: This emotional state involves a deep sense that the future holds no possibility for improvement. Individuals may feel that their circumstances will never change or that their actions cannot influence outcomes. Such beliefs often accompany severe depressive states. The perception of a meaningless future can intensify emotional distress. It may also increase risk for self-harm if the individual believes nothing can improve. Assessment of this emotional experience is essential during mental health evaluations. Treatment focuses on restoring hope through therapy and appropriate medication.

Q617. Answer: D

Explanation: This test assesses the ability to retain and recall information after a short delay. The task measures memory processes responsible for storing new information for brief periods. It evaluates whether the brain can encode, store, and retrieve recently learned data. Difficulty recalling words after a short delay may indicate impairment in memory processing. Such deficits may appear in several neurological or psychiatric conditions. Memory testing helps clinicians identify potential cognitive disorders. Results guide further evaluation and treatment planning.

Q618. Answer: A

Explanation: This condition involves a chronic form of depressed mood lasting for an extended period. Although symptoms may be less severe than those of major depressive episodes, they persist for years. Individuals often describe a constant low mood and reduced enjoyment of activities. Despite these feelings, they may continue to perform daily responsibilities. The prolonged nature of the symptoms distinguishes it from shorter depressive episodes. The disorder can significantly affect overall quality of life. Treatment typically involves psychotherapy combined with antidepressant medication.

Q619. Answer: C

Explanation: This rare but life-threatening reaction involves severe disruption of the body's temperature and muscle control systems. The condition develops when dopamine activity is significantly blocked by certain medications. Individuals may present with high fever, muscle rigidity, and altered mental status. Autonomic instability can cause fluctuating blood pressure and heart rate. Without immediate treatment, complications such as organ failure may occur. Prompt recognition is critical for patient safety. Treatment involves discontinuing the medication and providing intensive supportive care.

Q620. Answer: A

Explanation: This anxiety condition involves fear of situations where leaving or obtaining help might be difficult during distress. Crowded environments, public transportation, or large open areas may trigger anxiety. Individuals may avoid these places to prevent potential panic-like experiences. Over time, avoidance behaviors can significantly restrict daily activities. The fear often develops after experiencing anxiety in similar settings. The condition can lead to isolation if untreated. Therapy and medication can help reduce anxiety and restore normal functioning.

Q621. Answer: C

Explanation: This belief reflects the interpretation that ordinary events or communications contain special messages directed personally toward the individual. The person assigns personal significance to neutral external events. Media broadcasts, conversations, or random environmental cues may be perceived as coded signals meant specifically for them. The conviction persists despite evidence that the information is general and not personalized. Such beliefs can lead to confusion and distress as the individual attempts to interpret these perceived messages. This pattern is commonly observed in certain psychotic disorders. Treatment generally involves addressing the underlying condition through antipsychotic medication and therapeutic support.

Q622. Answer: C

Explanation: This pattern involves overinclusion of irrelevant or unnecessary details in conversation. The individual eventually returns to the original topic but only after lengthy explanations. The thought process remains logically connected but overly elaborate. Listeners may feel that the response is overly complicated or indirect. This style of communication can occur in several psychiatric conditions. It differs from disorganized thought because the individual ultimately answers the question. Recognition of this pattern helps clinicians better interpret patient communication.

Q623. Answer: D

Explanation: This phenomenon occurs when the flow of thinking suddenly stops without warning. The individual may pause during speech and appear confused or unable to continue their statement. After the interruption, they may not remember what they were discussing. This disruption reflects an interruption in the normal thought process. It may occur in several psychiatric conditions affecting cognition. The sudden halt in thinking can disrupt communication and concentration. Clinical assessment helps determine underlying causes and appropriate treatment.

Q624. Answer: A

Explanation: This experience involves a sense of separation from one's own body or mental processes. Individuals may feel as if they are watching themselves from an external perspective. The experience can be unsettling but the person usually recognizes that the sensation is unusual. It often occurs during periods of intense stress or anxiety. The perception reflects a disturbance in self-awareness rather than a loss of reality testing. Although distressing, individuals generally maintain insight about the experience. Treatment focuses on managing underlying anxiety or stress.

Q625. Answer: A

Explanation: This belief reflects an exaggerated sense of personal importance or abilities. Individuals may believe they possess exceptional talents, wealth, or influence. The conviction often persists despite evidence contradicting the claim. Such ideas can affect judgment and decision-making. The person may attempt actions based on the belief in these abilities. These beliefs are typically resistant to logical correction. Treatment focuses on reducing psychotic symptoms and improving insight.

Q626. Answer: D

Explanation: This condition results from excessive accumulation of serotonin in the central nervous system. The syndrome typically occurs when multiple medications that increase serotonin are combined. Symptoms may include agitation, sweating, tremor, confusion, and muscle rigidity. Autonomic instability may also develop, leading to rapid heart rate or changes in blood pressure. The condition can progress quickly if not recognized early. Immediate medical evaluation is necessary to prevent complications. Treatment involves discontinuing the offending agents and providing supportive care.

Q627. Answer: D

Explanation: This symptom refers to the diminished ability to experience pleasure from normally enjoyable activities. Individuals may lose interest in hobbies, social interactions, or previously rewarding experiences. The change often contributes to social withdrawal and reduced motivation. It is frequently observed in depressive disorders and some psychotic conditions. Emotional responsiveness may appear flattened or absent. The experience can significantly affect quality of life and interpersonal relationships. Treatment focuses on addressing the underlying mood disorder.

Q628. Answer: D

Explanation: This behavior involves the involuntary repetition of words or phrases spoken by another person. The repetition may occur immediately after hearing the words. It reflects a disturbance in normal communication patterns. The behavior can occur in several neurological or psychiatric conditions. The individual may not be intentionally copying the speech. Instead, the repetition occurs automatically. Recognition of this pattern can assist clinicians in identifying underlying disorders.

Q629. Answer: A

Explanation: This condition involves significant disturbances in motor behavior and responsiveness. Individuals may remain motionless for long periods or maintain unusual postures. They may show minimal reaction to external stimulation. Speech may be absent or extremely limited. The condition may occur in association with mood disorders or psychotic conditions. Without treatment, the individual may develop complications related to immobility. Prompt recognition allows clinicians to initiate appropriate therapeutic interventions.

Q630. Answer: A

Explanation: This pattern involves rapid transitions from one idea to another with understandable connections between topics. The individual may speak quickly and appear highly energized. Although ideas are connected, the conversation may become difficult to follow due to speed. The pattern often reflects heightened mental activity. It commonly appears during periods of elevated mood states. Listeners may feel overwhelmed by the rapid pace of ideas. Recognition of this pattern assists clinicians in identifying mood disturbances.

Q631. Answer: D

Explanation: This anxiety condition involves intense fear related to social interactions or performance situations. Individuals worry that others will evaluate them negatively. The fear may lead to avoidance of public speaking, group interactions, or meeting unfamiliar people. Physical symptoms such as sweating or trembling may accompany the anxiety. The distress can interfere with education, work, or relationships. Despite recognizing that the fear may be excessive, individuals struggle to control it. Treatment often includes psychotherapy and medications that reduce anxiety symptoms.

Q632. Answer: C

Explanation: This behavior represents a repetitive action performed to relieve anxiety associated with intrusive thoughts. Individuals may feel compelled to perform the action even when they recognize it as unnecessary. The behavior temporarily reduces distress but reinforces the cycle of anxiety and repetition. Over time, the ritual may become increasingly time-consuming. The underlying thoughts often involve fear of harm or catastrophe if the behavior is not performed. Such patterns are characteristic of certain anxiety-related conditions. Treatment focuses on interrupting the cycle through therapy and medication.

Q633. Answer: A

Explanation: This condition involves an acute disturbance in awareness and cognitive functioning. Individuals may have difficulty focusing attention or maintaining coherent thinking. The symptoms typically develop rapidly and fluctuate throughout the day. Disorientation and confusion are common features. Underlying medical conditions or substance use frequently contribute to the disorder. Prompt identification is essential because the condition may indicate serious medical problems. Treatment focuses on addressing the underlying cause and stabilizing cognitive function.

Q634. Answer: A

Explanation: This condition involves instability in emotional regulation, relationships, and self-image. Individuals may experience rapid shifts between admiration and anger toward others. Feelings of emptiness and fear of abandonment are common. Emotional responses can be intense and unpredictable. Impulsive behaviors may occur during periods of distress. Interpersonal relationships often become turbulent due to these emotional fluctuations. Psychotherapy focusing on emotional regulation and interpersonal effectiveness is commonly used in treatment.

Q635. Answer: B

Explanation: This condition involves ongoing difficulty initiating or maintaining sleep. Individuals may feel fatigued yet struggle to fall asleep even when given adequate opportunity. The lack of restorative sleep can impair daytime functioning. Concentration, mood, and energy levels may decline. The disorder may be influenced by stress, medical conditions, or behavioral factors. Over time, worry about sleep itself can worsen the problem. Treatment may include behavioral interventions and sleep hygiene strategies.

Q636. Answer: D

Explanation: This condition involves recurrent urges to pull out one's own hair. The behavior often occurs in response to tension or emotional distress. Individuals may feel temporary relief or satisfaction after pulling hair. Over time, repeated behavior may result in visible hair loss. The individual may attempt to hide the effects through hairstyles or clothing. The behavior is not related to a medical dermatologic condition. Treatment often includes behavioral therapy aimed at controlling impulses.

Q637. Answer: B

Explanation: This belief involves a false conviction related to bodily sensations or physical health. Individuals may insist that parasites, diseases, or bodily abnormalities exist despite normal examinations. The belief persists even when medical professionals provide clear evidence to the contrary. The person may repeatedly seek medical testing or treatment. The conviction reflects a distortion in the perception of bodily functioning. These beliefs often occur within certain psychiatric conditions involving psychosis. Treatment focuses on addressing the underlying disorder.

Q638. Answer: D

Explanation: This behavior involves the creation of entirely new words that are not recognized in the common language. The individual may assign unique meanings to these invented terms. Such speech patterns often reflect disruptions in thought organization. Listeners may find the communication confusing or difficult to interpret. The words are typically not understood by others without explanation. This pattern is commonly observed in certain psychotic disorders. Identification of unusual speech patterns can aid in psychiatric assessment.

Q639. Answer: B

Explanation: This pattern involves awakening earlier than desired and being unable to resume sleep. It is commonly associated with mood disorders, particularly depressive conditions. Individuals may feel exhausted yet unable to return to rest. The disruption contributes to fatigue and reduced daytime functioning. Sleep disturbances are important diagnostic clues in mental health assessment. Addressing the underlying mood disorder often improves sleep patterns. Treatment may include psychotherapy, medication, and sleep regulation strategies.

Q640. Answer: D

Explanation: This condition involves a longstanding pattern of violating social norms and the rights of others. Individuals may engage in deceitful or manipulative behavior for personal gain. Impulsivity and lack of remorse are common features. The person may disregard safety or legal boundaries. Relationships are often unstable due to exploitation of others. These behaviors typically begin in adolescence and continue into adulthood. Treatment focuses on behavioral interventions and structured therapeutic approaches.

Q641. Answer: B

Explanation: This condition involves persistent patterns of inattention and hyperactivity that interfere with daily functioning. Individuals may struggle to maintain focus on tasks or conversations. They often act impulsively and have difficulty remaining still during situations requiring sustained attention. These symptoms typically begin in childhood but may continue into adulthood. Problems with organization and task completion are common. The disorder can affect academic, occupational, and social performance. Treatment often includes behavioral strategies and medications that improve attention regulation.

Q642. Answer: B

Explanation: This disorder involves excessive daytime sleepiness and sudden uncontrollable episodes of sleep. Individuals may fall asleep unexpectedly during routine activities. The condition results from disruption of normal sleep-wake regulation in the brain. Some individuals may also experience sudden loss of muscle tone triggered by strong emotions. Sleep episodes can occur even after adequate nighttime rest. These symptoms significantly interfere with daily functioning. Management often involves medication and strategies to regulate sleep patterns.

Q643. Answer: A

Explanation: This condition involves an inability to recall important autobiographical information. The memory loss often occurs after a traumatic or stressful event. The individual remains conscious and aware but cannot retrieve specific memories. Unlike neurological memory disorders, the disturbance is psychological in origin. The memory gaps may involve specific events or periods of time. This mechanism may serve as a psychological defense against overwhelming stress. Treatment focuses on psychotherapy and emotional processing of the stressor.

Q644. Answer: D

Explanation: This disorder involves persistent worry about having or developing a serious medical condition. Individuals frequently seek reassurance from healthcare providers despite normal examinations. The fear remains strong even when test results confirm good health. Anxiety about health often leads to repeated checking of bodily sensations. The individual may misinterpret normal physical sensations as signs of illness. This pattern can significantly interfere with daily life. Treatment focuses on managing health-related anxiety through therapy and education.

Q645. Answer: C

Explanation: This anxiety condition involves intense fear triggered by a specific object or situation. Exposure to the feared stimulus may provoke immediate anxiety or panic. Individuals often avoid situations where they might encounter the trigger. The fear is usually recognized as excessive but remains difficult to control. Avoidance behaviors can limit normal activities and experiences. The condition often begins during childhood or adolescence. Treatment commonly includes exposure-based therapy and anxiety management techniques.

Q646. Answer: C

Explanation: This experience involves a perception that the external world feels strange or unreal. Individuals may describe their surroundings as foggy, distorted, or dreamlike. Although the sensation is disturbing, the person usually recognizes that the environment has not actually changed. The experience often occurs during intense stress or anxiety. It reflects a temporary disruption in normal perception of reality. Unlike psychosis, the individual typically maintains insight. Treatment focuses on managing stress and underlying anxiety.

Q647. Answer: B
Explanation: This pattern involves the inappropriate repetition of a word, phrase, or response. The repetition occurs even when the topic of conversation changes. It reflects difficulty shifting thoughts or responses to new stimuli. The behavior may occur in several neurological or psychiatric conditions. Communication may become repetitive and less meaningful over time. Observing this pattern can provide clues about cognitive functioning. Further assessment helps identify the underlying disorder.
Q648. Answer: A
Explanation: This condition involves recurrent urges to steal objects that are not needed for personal use or financial gain. The behavior is driven by increasing tension before the act and relief afterward. Individuals often feel guilt or embarrassment following the behavior. The stolen items may be discarded or hidden rather than used. The behavior is not motivated by anger or revenge. Instead, it reflects difficulty controlling impulses. Treatment often involves psychotherapy focused on impulse control.
Q649. Answer: A
Explanation: This episode involves a sustained period of abnormally elevated or irritable mood. Individuals may experience increased energy and reduced need for sleep. Their confidence may become exaggerated, leading to unrealistic beliefs about abilities. Risky behaviors such as impulsive spending or reckless decisions may occur. The disturbance often causes significant impairment in social or occupational functioning. In severe cases, hospitalization may be required to ensure safety. Treatment generally includes mood stabilizers and antipsychotic medications.
Q650. Answer: B
Explanation: This condition involves neurological symptoms that cannot be explained by a medical disorder. The symptoms may affect movement, sensation, or coordination. Psychological stress often precedes the onset of physical symptoms. The individual does not intentionally produce the symptoms. Instead, the symptoms represent an unconscious response to emotional conflict. Medical testing typically shows normal physiological functioning. Treatment focuses on addressing psychological stress and improving coping mechanisms.
Q651. Answer: B
Explanation: This belief reflects the conviction that one's private thoughts are accessible to others. The individual may feel that their mind is no longer private. They might believe others can hear or detect their thoughts without verbal expression. The belief persists even when there is no evidence supporting it. Such experiences often produce significant distress and social withdrawal. This symptom is commonly associated with certain psychotic disorders. Treatment focuses on reducing psychotic symptoms through medication and therapy.
Q652. Answer: A
Explanation: This condition occurs when psychological stress manifests as physical neurological symptoms. The individual may lose speech, movement, or sensation without an identifiable medical cause. The symptoms are not intentionally produced or feigned. Instead, they represent unconscious expression of emotional conflict. The physical changes often appear suddenly after a stressful event. Medical examinations typically show normal neurological functioning. Treatment focuses on addressing underlying psychological stressors.
Q653. Answer: D
Explanation: This disorder involves excessive preoccupation with perceived physical imperfections. The flaws may be minor or not visible to others. Individuals may spend large amounts of time checking mirrors or attempting to hide the perceived defect. The concern often leads to distress and avoidance of social situations. The belief about the flaw may become strongly fixed over time. Daily functioning can be significantly impaired by the preoccupation. Treatment typically includes cognitive behavioral therapy and medication.
Q654. Answer: B

Explanation: This speech pattern is characterized by the use of words chosen for their sound rather than their meaning. Rhyming or alliteration may dominate the conversation. The words may appear connected phonetically but lack logical coherence. This pattern reflects disruption in organized thinking. Listeners may find the speech confusing or difficult to interpret. The behavior often appears in certain psychiatric conditions affecting thought processes. Recognition of abnormal speech patterns aids clinical assessment.

Q655. Answer: C

Explanation: This condition involves instability in relationships, emotional regulation, and self-image. Individuals often fear being abandoned by important people in their lives. Emotional responses may be intense and rapidly changing. Impulsive behaviors such as spending, substance use, or risky actions may occur during distress. Relationships often alternate between idealization and conflict. The emotional instability can significantly disrupt daily functioning. Psychotherapy focusing on emotional regulation is commonly used for treatment.

Q656. Answer: B

Explanation: This cognitive function involves the ability to focus mental resources on a specific task or stimulus. Individuals with impairment may struggle to maintain concentration. External stimuli such as noise or movement can easily disrupt focus. Attention is essential for learning, memory, and problem solving. Difficulty maintaining focus can affect many areas of daily functioning. Mental status examinations often include tasks that evaluate sustained attention. Identifying deficits helps clinicians assess neurological or psychiatric conditions.

Q657. Answer: B

Explanation: This anxiety condition involves excessive fear or distress when separated from attachment figures. The individual may worry about possible harm occurring to themselves or the loved one. Physical symptoms of anxiety may develop during separation. The person may resist being alone or away from the attachment figure. Although often associated with children, it can also occur in adults. The fear interferes with normal independence and daily functioning. Treatment may involve psychotherapy focused on managing anxiety and building coping skills.

Q658. Answer: B

Explanation: This behavior reflects repetitive actions performed to reduce anxiety associated with intrusive thoughts. Individuals may feel a strong urge to arrange objects in a specific order. Distress occurs if the pattern is disrupted or incomplete. The behavior temporarily relieves anxiety but reinforces the cycle over time. These rituals may become time-consuming and interfere with daily activities. The individual often recognizes that the behavior is excessive. Treatment frequently includes cognitive behavioral therapy and medications that affect serotonin regulation.

Q659. Answer: D

Explanation: This phenomenon occurs during the transition between sleep and wakefulness. Individuals may be conscious but unable to move their muscles temporarily. Vivid visual or auditory hallucinations may accompany the experience. The episodes typically last a few seconds to minutes before normal movement returns. Although frightening, the condition is usually harmless. It often occurs during periods of disrupted sleep or stress. Improving sleep hygiene can reduce the frequency of episodes.

Q660. Answer: B

Explanation: This neurological condition involves repeated involuntary motor movements and sometimes vocalizations. The movements occur suddenly and may vary in frequency or intensity. Individuals often feel a buildup of tension before the movement occurs. Performing the movement may temporarily relieve the sensation. The symptoms usually begin during childhood. They may fluctuate over time but often persist into adulthood. Treatment focuses on behavioral therapy and medications that reduce tic frequency.

Q661. Answer: B

Explanation: This belief involves the conviction that others intend to harm, spy on, or conspire against the individual. The person may misinterpret ordinary actions of others as threatening or directed specifically toward them. These beliefs persist despite lack of supporting evidence. The perception of danger often leads to heightened suspicion and social withdrawal. Individuals may take defensive actions to protect themselves from perceived threats. Such beliefs are frequently associated with psychotic disorders. Treatment focuses on reducing psychotic symptoms and improving reality testing.

Q662. Answer: D

Explanation: This behavior represents a repetitive action performed to reduce anxiety caused by intrusive thoughts. The individual feels driven to perform the action even when recognizing it may be unnecessary. The ritual temporarily relieves distress but reinforces the underlying anxiety cycle. Over time the behavior may become increasingly time-consuming. Individuals may structure large parts of their routine around these behaviors. The pattern reflects an attempt to neutralize uncomfortable thoughts or fears. Treatment often involves therapy that helps break the cycle of anxiety and repetitive behavior.

Q663. Answer: B

Explanation: This mood state involves a period of abnormally elevated energy and activity levels. Individuals may feel unusually productive and confident during this time. Reduced need for sleep often accompanies the increased energy. People may begin numerous projects without completing them. Decision-making may become impulsive or risky due to heightened confidence. These episodes can significantly disrupt personal and occupational functioning. Proper treatment typically involves mood stabilizing medications and monitoring.

Q664. Answer: B

Explanation: This cognitive function involves the ability to understand concepts and relationships between ideas. Tasks requiring identification of similarities between objects assess abstract thinking. Individuals with impairment may focus on superficial or literal characteristics rather than conceptual connections. Abstract reasoning is important for problem solving and understanding complex ideas. Deficits may occur in several neurological or psychiatric conditions. Assessment helps clinicians evaluate higher-level cognitive functioning. Identifying impairment can guide further diagnostic evaluation.

Q665. Answer: D

Explanation: This condition involves significant distress related to physical symptoms that may or may not have a medical explanation. Individuals become excessively focused on bodily sensations. The concern leads to repeated healthcare visits and persistent worry. Even minor symptoms may be interpreted as serious health problems. The distress associated with the symptoms can impair daily functioning. Unlike some other conditions, the symptoms themselves are central to the concern. Treatment focuses on managing health anxiety and improving coping strategies.

Q666. Answer: C

Explanation: This anxiety disorder involves intense fear related to social or performance situations. Individuals worry that others will judge or criticize them negatively. Situations such as public speaking may provoke strong physical symptoms of anxiety. These symptoms may include sweating, trembling, or rapid heartbeat. Avoidance of feared situations often develops as a coping strategy. Over time the avoidance may interfere with academic or professional responsibilities. Treatment often involves cognitive behavioral therapy and anxiety-reducing medications.

Q667. Answer: B

Explanation: This condition involves significant abnormalities in motor behavior. Individuals may maintain unusual postures or remain immobile for extended periods. They may resist attempts by others to reposition them. Speech may be minimal or absent during episodes. The condition can occur in association with mood disorders or psychotic disorders. Without treatment, complications such as dehydration or muscle injury may occur. Recognition allows clinicians to initiate appropriate medical and psychiatric interventions.

Q668. Answer: D

Explanation: This experience involves a sudden surge of intense fear or discomfort. Physical symptoms often develop rapidly and peak within minutes. Individuals may feel as if they are losing control or experiencing a medical emergency. The episodes may occur unexpectedly and without warning. Although the symptoms are frightening, they typically resolve within a short time. Recurrent episodes can lead to ongoing anxiety about future attacks. Treatment focuses on managing anxiety and preventing recurrence.

Q669. Answer: B

Explanation: This personality pattern involves an inflated sense of self-importance and entitlement. Individuals often believe they deserve special recognition or privileges. They may exaggerate achievements or talents to gain admiration. Empathy toward others may be limited because attention remains focused on personal needs. Relationships can become strained due to expectations of admiration and validation. Criticism may provoke strong emotional reactions. Psychotherapy often focuses on developing empathy and realistic self-perception.

Q670. Answer: B

Explanation: This condition occurs when psychological stress manifests as neurological symptoms. Individuals may develop weakness, paralysis, or sensory disturbances without a medical cause. The symptoms are not intentionally produced. Instead, they represent an unconscious response to emotional conflict. Medical examinations typically show normal neurological functioning. The symptoms often appear shortly after a stressful event. Treatment focuses on addressing underlying psychological stressors and improving coping strategies.

Q671. Answer: C

Explanation: This condition involves intrusive thoughts that create significant anxiety. Individuals attempt to reduce the distress by performing repetitive actions. Arranging objects in a specific order may become a ritual used to reduce anxiety. The behavior may provide temporary relief but reinforces the cycle of intrusive thoughts and compulsive actions. Over time the rituals may interfere with normal daily activities. Individuals usually recognize that the behaviors are excessive. Treatment commonly involves cognitive behavioral therapy and medication.

Q672. Answer: D

Explanation: This symptom involves hearing sounds or voices without any external auditory stimulus. The perception originates internally rather than from the environment. The voices may comment on the individual's actions or speak directly to them. These experiences often feel extremely real to the person. They can cause distress, fear, or difficulty concentrating. Such symptoms are frequently associated with psychotic disorders. Treatment focuses on addressing the underlying psychiatric condition.

Q673. Answer: B

Explanation: This condition involves recurrent urges to steal objects that are not needed for personal use. The behavior is driven by increasing tension before the act. After the act is completed, the individual may feel relief or satisfaction. Feelings of guilt or embarrassment often follow the behavior. The stolen items are typically not used or kept for personal value. The behavior reflects difficulty controlling impulses. Treatment often focuses on therapy aimed at improving impulse regulation.

Q674. Answer: A

Explanation: This cognitive function refers to awareness of time, place, and personal identity. Orientation helps individuals understand where they are and what is happening around them. Disorientation may cause confusion about the current date, location, or situation. Such impairment can occur in neurological conditions or acute medical illnesses. Assessment of orientation is a standard component of mental status examinations. Identifying deficits helps clinicians evaluate cognitive functioning. Treatment depends on addressing the underlying cause of the impairment.

Q675. Answer: D

Explanation: This belief involves a fixed false idea concerning bodily sensations or functions. Individuals may believe that they have a physical abnormality despite lack of evidence. The conviction persists even after medical evaluation confirms normal findings. Such beliefs often cause embarrassment or social avoidance. The person may attempt to conceal or repeatedly check the perceived problem. These beliefs may occur in several psychiatric conditions. Treatment focuses on managing the underlying disorder and improving insight.

Q676. Answer: A

Explanation: This sleep disorder involves repeated pauses in breathing during sleep. These interruptions reduce oxygen levels and disrupt normal sleep cycles. Individuals may wake frequently during the night without fully realizing it. As a result, they experience excessive daytime fatigue and difficulty concentrating. Loud snoring and morning headaches are also common. The condition can increase risk for cardiovascular problems if untreated. Treatment often includes devices that help maintain airway patency during sleep.

Q677. Answer: D

Explanation: This condition involves an acute disturbance in attention and awareness. Symptoms often develop quickly over hours or days. Individuals may appear confused, disoriented, and unable to focus on tasks. The severity of symptoms often fluctuates throughout the day. Medical conditions such as infections commonly trigger the disturbance. Early recognition is important because the condition may indicate serious underlying illness. Treatment focuses on addressing the medical cause and stabilizing cognitive function.

Q678. Answer: C

Explanation: This behavior represents a repetitive action performed to relieve anxiety associated with intrusive thoughts. Individuals feel driven to perform the action even when recognizing it may not be logical. The act temporarily reduces distress but reinforces the underlying pattern. The cycle of anxiety and repetitive behavior may become increasingly rigid. Individuals often attempt to resist the urge but feel unable to do so. Such behaviors are characteristic of certain anxiety-related conditions. Treatment focuses on breaking the cycle through therapy and medication.

Q679. Answer: C

Explanation: This mood disorder involves persistent sadness and diminished interest in daily activities. Individuals may experience fatigue, sleep disturbances, and difficulty concentrating. Emotional symptoms often interfere with work, relationships, and personal responsibilities. Feelings of hopelessness or guilt may also occur. The symptoms typically last for several weeks or longer. Early recognition is important because untreated depression can significantly affect quality of life. Treatment often includes psychotherapy and antidepressant medications.

Q680. Answer: A

Explanation: This personality pattern involves excessive reliance on others for guidance and support. Individuals may struggle to make decisions without reassurance. They often fear abandonment and feel uncomfortable when alone. The need for care may lead them to tolerate unhealthy relationships. Self-confidence is typically low and independence is limited. The behavior pattern often begins in early adulthood. Psychotherapy focuses on building self-confidence and decision-making abilities.

Q681. Answer: A

Explanation: Trichotillomania is characterized by recurrent hair pulling that results in hair loss. The behavior is usually triggered by stress, tension, or anxiety. Individuals may feel increasing urge before pulling the hair and relief afterward. Hair may be pulled from the scalp, eyebrows, or other body areas. The behavior can lead to embarrassment and social withdrawal. It is classified among obsessive-compulsive related disorders. Treatment often involves behavioral therapy and sometimes medication.

Q682. Answer: B

Explanation: A referential delusion occurs when individuals believe that neutral events or messages are specifically directed toward them. The person misinterprets ordinary occurrences such as media broadcasts or conversations as having special meaning. These beliefs persist even when others explain the situation logically. The interpretation is strongly fixed and resistant to evidence. Such delusions are often associated with psychotic disorders. They may cause anxiety or suspicious behavior. Treatment focuses on reducing psychotic symptoms and improving insight.

Q683. Answer: D

Explanation: Nihilistic delusions involve the false belief that oneself, others, or the world no longer exists. Individuals may believe that their body is decaying or that life has ended. These beliefs are often associated with severe depression or psychotic conditions. The person may appear hopeless or detached from reality. Such beliefs can significantly increase risk of self-harm. Immediate psychiatric evaluation is usually required. Treatment includes medication and supportive therapy.

Q684. Answer: C

Explanation: Dissociative fugue involves sudden travel away from one's home combined with inability to recall personal identity. The individual may appear normal to others during the episode. Memory loss is usually related to severe stress or trauma. The person may assume a new identity temporarily. Once the episode ends, confusion about events that occurred during the fugue may remain. The condition reflects disruption in normal memory and identity integration. Treatment focuses on psychotherapy and stress management.

Q685. Answer: D

Explanation: Depersonalization refers to a feeling of detachment from one's own body or mental processes. Individuals may feel as if they are observing themselves from outside. Despite the unusual experience, they typically recognize that the sensation is not real. The episodes may occur during periods of intense stress or anxiety. Perception of reality remains intact. These experiences can be frightening but are not psychotic. Treatment often focuses on reducing anxiety and improving coping mechanisms.

Q686. Answer: B

Explanation: Generalized anxiety disorder involves excessive worry about multiple aspects of daily life. The anxiety is difficult to control and occurs on most days. Physical symptoms such as fatigue, muscle tension, and restlessness often accompany the worry. The condition may interfere with concentration and sleep. Individuals may anticipate negative outcomes even in routine situations. Symptoms typically persist for at least six months. Treatment includes cognitive behavioral therapy and medication.

Q687. Answer: B

Explanation: During manic episodes individuals often experience a decreased need for sleep. They may feel energetic and active despite minimal rest. Unlike insomnia, they do not feel tired during the day. Increased goal-directed activity often accompanies this symptom. The person may start many projects simultaneously. Judgment may become impaired due to excessive confidence. Mood stabilizing treatment is usually required.

Q688. Answer: B

Explanation: A compulsion is a repetitive behavior performed to relieve anxiety created by intrusive thoughts. The individual feels compelled to perform the action even when recognizing it may be unnecessary. Checking behaviors are common compulsions. The act temporarily reduces anxiety but reinforces the cycle. Over time the behavior may become time-consuming. These symptoms are commonly seen in obsessive-compulsive disorder. Treatment focuses on therapy aimed at reducing compulsive rituals.

Q689. Answer: D

Explanation: Grandiose delusions involve exaggerated beliefs about one's importance, abilities, or identity. Individuals may believe they have unique talents or a special purpose. These beliefs are not supported by reality but remain firmly held. The person may expect admiration or special treatment from others. Such delusions may appear in mania or psychotic disorders. They can lead to risky or unrealistic behavior. Treatment focuses on stabilizing mood and reducing psychotic symptoms.

Q690. Answer: D

Explanation: A hallucination is a sensory perception that occurs without an external stimulus. Visual hallucinations involve seeing objects or images that are not present. The experience may feel completely real to the individual. These symptoms may occur in psychiatric disorders, substance use, or neurological conditions. The content of hallucinations varies widely. Such experiences can be distressing or frightening. Treatment depends on addressing the underlying cause.

Q691. Answer: D

Explanation: A specific phobia involves intense fear of a particular object or situation. Elevators, animals, or heights are common triggers. The fear is usually disproportionate to the actual danger involved. Individuals may go to great lengths to avoid the feared situation. Exposure to the trigger often produces immediate anxiety. The avoidance may interfere with daily activities. Behavioral therapy is commonly used in treatment.

Q692. Answer: C

Explanation: Short-term memory involves retaining information for brief periods. Difficulty remembering recent events indicates impairment in this type of memory. Individuals may repeatedly ask the same questions or forget recent instructions. Long-term memories such as childhood events may remain intact. Short-term memory problems are common in certain neurological conditions. Assessment helps determine the severity of cognitive impairment. Treatment focuses on addressing underlying causes and supporting memory function.

Q693. Answer: C

Explanation: Antisocial personality disorder involves persistent disregard for social rules and the rights of others. Individuals may engage in deceitful or reckless behaviors. Lack of empathy and remorse is a common feature. Such individuals may manipulate others for personal gain. The behavior pattern often begins in adolescence. Relationships and occupational stability are frequently affected. Treatment focuses on behavioral management and long-term therapy.

Q694. Answer: A

Explanation: Post-traumatic stress disorder develops after exposure to a traumatic event. Individuals may experience intrusive memories, flashbacks, or nightmares related to the trauma. They often avoid reminders of the event. Hyperarousal symptoms such as irritability and difficulty sleeping may occur. The symptoms persist for more than one month. The condition can significantly disrupt daily functioning. Treatment includes trauma-focused therapy and medication.

Q695. Answer: A

Explanation: Misinterpretation of social cues occurs when individuals incorrectly perceive neutral behaviors as negative or threatening. This distortion may contribute to interpersonal conflicts. People may assume others are criticizing or rejecting them without evidence. Such interpretations often increase anxiety or anger. This pattern may appear in several psychiatric conditions. Cognitive therapy can help individuals reevaluate these perceptions. Improving social understanding often reduces emotional distress.

Q696. Answer: A

Explanation: Burnout syndrome occurs when prolonged stress leads to emotional and physical exhaustion. Individuals may feel overwhelmed and unable to cope with work demands. Motivation and productivity often decline. Concentration problems and fatigue are common symptoms. The condition may also lead to irritability and reduced job satisfaction. Without intervention, mental health problems may develop. Management includes stress reduction and lifestyle adjustments.

Q697. Answer: A

Explanation: Thought control delusion occurs when individuals believe that their thoughts are being manipulated by outside forces. They may feel that someone else is controlling their mind. This belief persists despite evidence to the contrary. Such symptoms are common in certain psychotic disorders. The experience can cause fear or loss of personal identity. Treatment focuses on managing psychotic symptoms. Antipsychotic medications are often used.

Q698. Answer: A

Explanation: Thought blocking occurs when a person suddenly stops speaking because the train of thought disappears. The pause may last several seconds or longer. When speech resumes, the individual may start a completely different topic. This disturbance reflects interruption in normal thought processes. It is often observed in psychotic disorders. The experience may feel confusing to the individual. Treatment focuses on managing the underlying psychiatric condition.

Q699. Answer: A

Explanation: Flight of ideas involves rapid shifting from one idea to another. Although connections between ideas may exist, they are often superficial. Speech may appear pressured and difficult to interrupt. This pattern commonly occurs during manic episodes. The individual may struggle to maintain focus on a single topic. Listeners may find the conversation difficult to follow. Treatment focuses on stabilizing mood and reducing manic symptoms.

Q700. Answer: B

Explanation: Insight refers to the individual's awareness and understanding of their own mental condition. Lack of insight occurs when a person does not recognize that they are experiencing psychological problems. This can interfere with willingness to seek or accept treatment. The individual may attribute symptoms to external factors instead. Poor insight is common in several psychiatric disorders. Assessment of insight helps clinicians plan appropriate interventions. Treatment may involve education and supportive therapy.

Made in the USA
Monee, IL
05 November 2026

67979980R00125